THE ART OF
INDIAN
HEAD MASSAGE

FOR RICHARD, EMMA AND LIZZIE – WITH ALL MY LOVE

THIS IS A CARLTON BOOK

First published by Carlton Books Limited, 2000.
This edition published in 2011.

10 9 8 7 6 5 4 3 2 1

Text © Mary Atkinson, 2000
Design © Carlton Books Limited, 2000

A CIP catalogue record for this book is available from the
British Library

ISBN: 978 1 84732 746 8

Project Editor Camilla MacWhannell
Project Art Direction Trevor Newman
Jacket Design Jake da'Costa
Design Simon Mercer
Picture Research Alex Pepper
Production Garry Lewis

Printed and bound in China

THE ART OF
INDIAN
HEAD MASSAGE

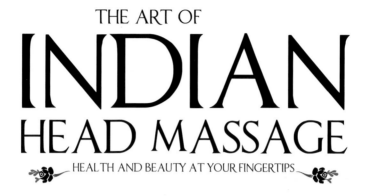

HEALTH AND BEAUTY AT YOUR FINGERTIPS

MARY ATKINSON

CARLTON
BOOKS

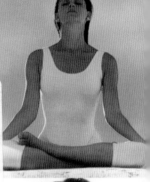

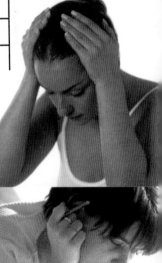

Contents

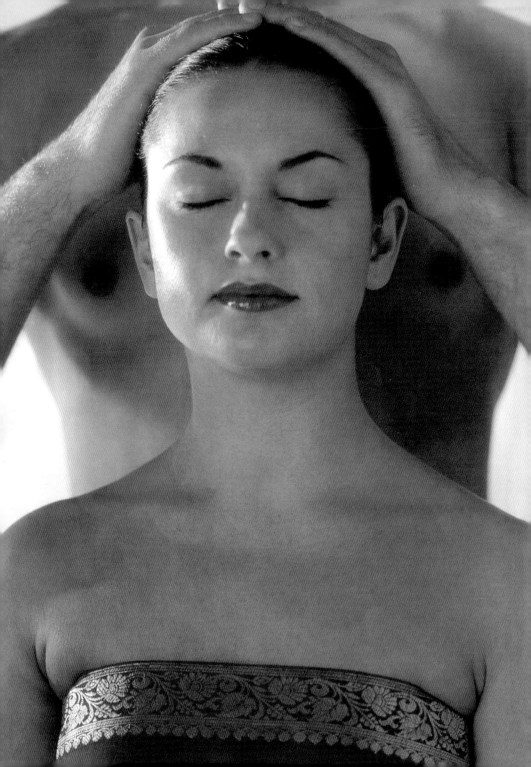

Introduction

INDIAN HEAD MASSAGE is as pleasurable to give as it is to receive. As you begin to practise the techniques on your family and friends, you should find this ancient art to be calming, revitalizing, uplifting and incredibly rewarding. Much of the joy lies in its simplicity, effectiveness and accessibility – no special equipment is needed and it takes less than half an hour to complete. With a few basic strokes, you can relax and soothe or invigorate and stimulate. It is a wonderful way of pacifying a troubled child to sleep, refreshing a jaded computer-user or pampering your loved ones with some tender loving care. You can also continue a long tradition followed by Indian women, men and children and enjoy head massage to give hair a healthy, lustrous shine.

Indian head massage not only works on the scalp, as the name suggests, but also on the face, shoulders, upper back and arms. These are all areas where we tend to harbour a great deal of tension, perhaps arising from poor posture, an accumulation of emotional stress, or spending long periods in front of a computer screen. The various different movements can help to relax taut and uncomfortable muscles, ease stiffness, stimulate the blood circulation and drain away excess toxins, so helping to relieve headaches and eye strain and increase joint mobility. Indian head massage also encourages deeper breathing and helps boost the flow of freshly oxygenated blood to the brain, resulting in more focused thought, greater concentration and better memory.

In the hurly-burly of everyday activities, we often deprive ourselves of the opportunity to be still and quiet and to simply "be ourselves". An Indian head massage can provide the incentive to switch off from any spiralling worries and hassles and centre yourself on the "here and now". This healing period in the day allows time for a busy mind to rest and recuperate and enables you to look at life from a new perspective. People emerge from the blissful experience of deep relaxation with renewed vigour, creativity and sense of purpose. It is an exhilarating yet peaceful feeling, often described as relaxed awareness, that brings the manifold benefits of more restful sleep, increased energy and vitality, and relief from stress and mild depression.

Regular Indian head massage can also improve the condition of your hair and skin, resulting in a generally younger, fresher and more attractive appearance. An efficient blood and lymph circulation ensures the living cells of the hair and skin are provided with fresh supplies of oxygen and nutrients and that any toxic residues are speedily removed from the body, thereby ensuring healthy growth and functioning. Nourishing oils have a cleansing, moisturizing and strengthening effect and can protect hair and skin from the harmful effects of the elements, pollution and general wear and tear.

Indian head massage does not diagnose or cure, but promotes the mental and physical conditions necessary to foster positive good health and prevent ill health.

Above all, Indian head massage is an exquisitely enjoyable sensation that triggers the release in the body of "feel good" chemicals called endorphins, creating an almost euphoric sensation of contentment and happiness. Much of the pleasure comes from the shared experience of an affectionate touch. Touch is a powerful and instinctive way of creating a bond that can communicate empathy far more effectively than words. Giving and receiving close, nurturing physical contact in a caring situation is one of our most basic human needs – and one that we tend to neglect, often without realizing it. People who have spent a period of time in isolation talk of the devastating effects of deprivation, not only of social contact but also of the caring touch of family and friends. You will find that the mutual enjoyment of an Indian head massage can strengthen relationships, boost morale and make the world seem a far better place.

The Art of Indian Head Massage has been written to help you share the pleasure of this ancient therapy safely and effectively with your family and friends. It is not a substitute for formal teaching but will introduce you to some of the basic techniques and encourage you to develop your own special style of massage. As you will soon discover, part of the fascination of Indian head massage is that no two massages are ever the same. Use your imagination to have fun experimenting with different strokes, devising your own routines to suit your partner and blending oils to make each individual massage a unique experience. Be creative – and focus your thoughts on enjoying the moment.

Mary Atkinson

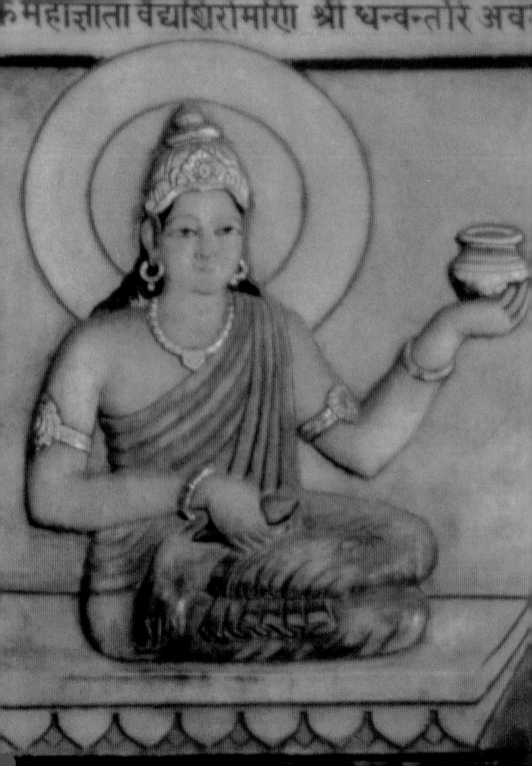

ऊं महाज्ञाता वैद्याशिरोमाणे श्री धन्वन्तरे अव

CHAPTER ONE

AN ANCIENT ART IN A MODERN WORLD

I NDIAN HEAD MASSAGE has a long and colourful history. It is based on a traditional system of medicine known as Ayurveda, which has been practised in India for over three thousand years and is becoming increasingly popular in the West. The word "Ayurveda" comes from Sanskrit, the ancient language of India, and means "science of life" or "knowledge of life". Ayurveda is a complete healing system, possibly the oldest in the world, which teaches a truly holistic approach, concentrating on achieving a balance of mind, body and spirit to promote physical, emotional and spiritual health and well-being.

The origins of Indian head massage

According to the Ayurvedic system, there are five fundamental elements in all living things – air, fire, water, earth and ether – that are forever changing and interacting. These are represented in the human body by three vital energies, or forces, known as "doshas", which are individually called vata, pitta and kapha. The level of these doshas within the body is influenced by certain foods, varying temperatures, times of day, levels of stress and many other factors. In their normal balanced state, the doshas provide strength and govern the normal functioning of bodily systems. An imbalance of the doshas leads to disease, illness and unhappiness.

Ayurveda works on the philosophy that each person is a unique entity with her own specific balance and combination of doshas. A trained Ayurvedic practitioner asks many detailed questions and performs various tests, such as taking the pulse and examining the tongue. The practitioner seeks to establish the patient's particular doshic constitution and find any imbalances before prescribing medication or other treatments. However, most of us have one or two dominant doshas that can be readily identified.

In general terms, vatas tend to be slightly built with dry skin and hair, fluctuating moods, a creative mind and a tendency toward insomnia and vivid dreams. Pittas are of medium build, with fair or medium colouring and fine, straight hair that has a tendency to go grey prematurely. They are usually efficient and ambitious with a good memory. Kaphas usually have smooth, oily skin, thick hair and find it hard to lose weight. They tend to be large, strong and rather lethargic with a caring and patient temperament.

A tailored lifestyle programme

An ideal lifestyle programme to maintain good health and prevent ill health is specified for each doshic constitution. What is good for one person may not be right for another. All aspects of health and well-being are covered by Ayurveda including diet, yoga, meditation, exercise, personal hygiene, internal cleansing, herbal remedies and massage with therapeutic oils. Although few modern families adhere to all the rituals and rules of a strictly authentic Ayurvedic way of life, the basic principles are followed in many homes and it remains the dominant system of health care in the Indian subcontinent.

The value of massage

Massage has long been an integral part of everyday life in India. According to Ayurvedic custom, a weekly massage is recommended for men and women to maintain a healthy balance of doshas and promote soft skin and strong, shiny hair. Before a wedding, the bride and groom are massaged with special oils to promote health, beauty and fertility. Women are massaged to help them cope with the physical and emotional strain of labour and, for forty days after the birth, new mothers and their babies receive a daily recuperative massage.

For Indian mothers, massage is regarded as an essential skill and an important means of communicating and bonding with their children, helping to create a secure and caring family atmosphere within the home. From the age of three or four, children receive from their mothers a daily

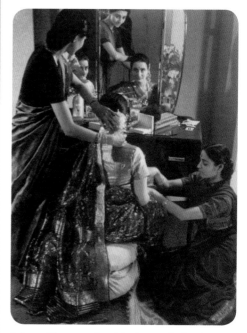

Indian wedding preparations. A head massage is often given prior to the big event to promote health, beauty and fertility.

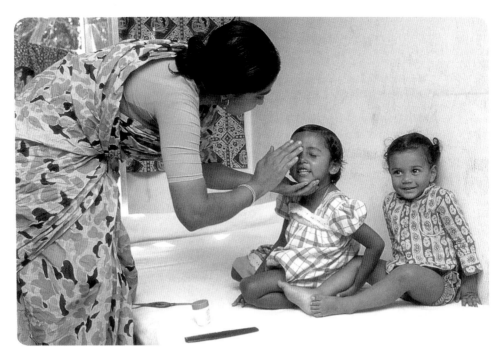

A woman from Calcutta moisturizes her daughter's face.

or weekly head massage, given with a selection of pungent oils, in the belief that this will help prevent scalp disorders, make their hair grow strong and also boost brain power. It is a custom that still holds fast, despite the fact that many youngsters, especially boys, rebel against being made to go out and play while they have oil on their heads. Many adults remark that it is only when they grow up and realize the benefits of regular head massage that they appreciate their mother's concern.

In the West, we tend to view the scalp as independent from the rest of the body and treat it in a different way. In India, however, the scalp is regarded as an extension of the body skin and lavished with the same care and attention. Most Indian women continue to massage their heads with nourishing oils and are rewarded with the long, vibrant, glossy hair that is much admired in Indian society. Mothers share suggestions for hair care and beauty routines with their daughters who, in turn, hand them down to their own offspring. There is no formal structure or set routine but, rather like a recipe that has been passed down through the generations, head massage has been developed and refined, with each region and family adding their own special touches to suit the climate, personalities and particular occasions.

☙ Oils and herbs

In India, a head massage is not complete without the use of ghee (clarified butter) or warm organic vegetable oils, chosen according to the season and availability within the region. These oils are often mixed with a selection of herbs, spices or fruits, such as amla (Indian gooseberry). Another popular ingredient is henna, a pale green powder from the dried shoots and leaves of the Lawsonia alba plant, which is used to dye and condition hair. Oils may be blended to a special family recipe or to alleviate a certain condition – perhaps to ease anxiety or moisturize a dry scalp. In Ayurvedic health centres, blends of oils and medicinal herbs are recommended to suit the dominant dosha. Vatas, for example, are generally advised to use a "warming" oil, such as sesame or mustard, as a base, whereas kaphas should choose a "cooling" oil, such as coconut or sunflower, mixed with herbal extracts. In some parts of India, women like to leave the oil on their heads for 24 hours or more, while others shampoo it off after a few hours.

Head massage has not remained an entirely female practice. Over the years, it has become incorporated into treatments offered to men by barbers and masseurs. It is believed that royalty and other eminent people used to employ personal head masseurs. There are even stories that these masseurs sometimes acted as spies who were able to draw out secrets while their clients were in the soporific state that can be induced by massage. Today, head massage is still included in any treatment provided by a barber, even a wet shave, and many men claim that it helps prevent early balding and greying – although this has not yet been scientifically proven.

Powerful touch

The massage generally performed in Ayurvedic health centres in India and usually offered to visitors tends to be extremely brisk and powerful. Although Indian masseurs may look very frail, their fingers can feel like rods of iron against your scalp. The massage is often too rough and vigorous for Westerners, who prefer a gentler touch. Many have vivid memories and claim "I thought my eyes were going to pop out of my head" or "It felt like my head was a spin drier" and "I was worried his fingers would go straight through my scalp". However, it must be added that these same people nearly always go on to extol the many benefits they derived from it, including deep relaxation, freedom from aches and pains, more restful sleep and better concentration.

A Western dimension

The concept of Indian head massage as a complementary therapy was first introduced into the UK by Dr Narendra Mehta, who arrived from India in the early 1970s to train as a physiotherapist. Like many Indian people away from their home country, he began to miss the benefits of a regular head massage and so decided it was time to develop it in the West. He returned to India to study different family and regional techniques and extended his particular style of scalp massage to include the neck, shoulders, upper back, upper arms and face. Balancing the flow of the body's subtle life energy – or "prana", as it is known in India – is an important part of Ayurveda and many other Eastern medical philosophies. Dr Mehta's form of Indian head massage, which he calls "champissage", also involves balancing the flow of energy by working on the body's energy centres – or "chakras" – a feature often included by trained therapists.

A chakra is believed to be a whirling vortex that draws energy into the body, allowing it to flow freely through the network of energy centres. The word "chakra" also comes from the ancient Sanskrit language and literally means "circle of movement". There are seven main chakras located at different levels, running from the master chakra on the crown of the head to the lowest one at the base of the spine.

CASE STUDY

Healthy hair

Saradha, 23, a trainee shop manager, moved from India when she was six years old. She follows her mother's and grandmother's example by giving herself a head massage every week to keep her long, dark hair strong and shiny. Sometimes her mother gives her a massage. "It is a lovely feeling when my mother tends my hair," she says. "She knows instinctively what mood I'm in and does a different kind of massage depending on how I'm feeling. When I'm tired and stressed, it is just so relaxing. I have tried using all sorts of different oils on my hair but I find that coconut is very light and easy to apply. It doesn't have

much smell, which is good as I like to sleep with the oil on my head. Some of the oils my mother prefers have such strong aromas that I would wake up with a migraine!

"While she massages my head, my mother tells me all about my early life in India. I love hearing the old stories about how children have their head massaged by their mothers and grandmothers. I haven't got any children yet but I would like to follow the tradition. My sisters massage their children's heads using the same kind of movements as my mother. But they don't sit still for long – just enough to get the oil into the hair and scalp!"

Therapists work with the chakras to release any stagnant energy within the body and restore a balance that brings a feeling of inner harmony and peace.

Indian head massage has become so popular that it is now widely taught at colleges in many parts of the world. It is enjoyed by people of all ages and walks of life and practised in a number of different settings, including private homes, natural health centres and hair and beauty salons. The massage has also been adapted so that it can be performed without oil, therefore clients do not need to disrobe and so the working day is not interrupted for long. As such, it has become firmly established as the ultimate antidote to the demands of modern life and is taken into offices, schools, hospices and even airports to help reduce tension, ease anxiety, increase clarity of thought and promote positive health and well-being.

An Indian head massage is now becoming a popular way to release tension and promote well-being in the work place.

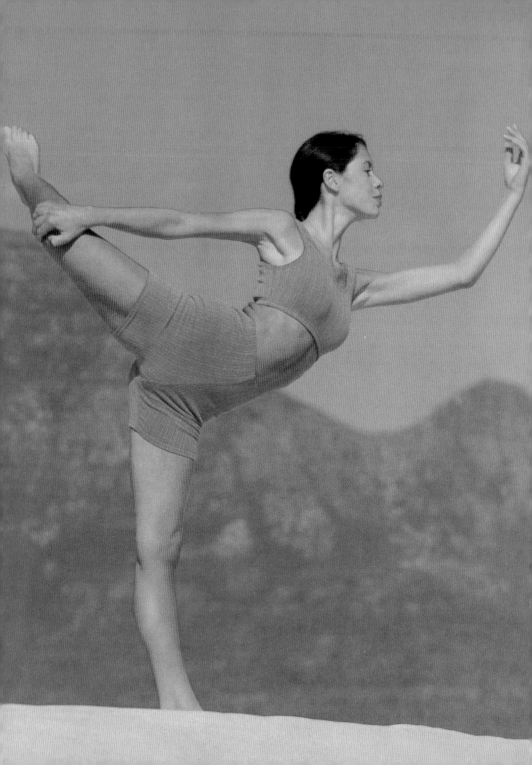

CHAPTER TWO

HEALTHY BODY, HEALTHY MIND

ABASIC KNOWLEDGE of how Indian head massage affects some of the main structures and systems of the body can help you to appreciate the benefits of the therapy and enable you to give a more effective and personal massage. As you start to realize the amazing intricacies of the miraculous body machine, you will develop a greater understanding of the impact of the various different techniques and learn how to adapt your sequence of movements to meet the individual needs of your massage partner.

✆ Therapeutic effects

This chapter looks at the blood and lymph circulation, the musculoskeletal system, skin and hair, and the effect of stress on our lives. When studying aspects of anatomy and physiology, however, it is important not to regard any mental or physical system in total isolation. Everything within the mind and body is inter-linked and interacts so that an imbalance in one system can have a profound effect on your overall health and well-being.

✆ Life-giving blood

Blood is the body's main transport system. It distributes vital supplies of oxygen and nutrients to the billions of living cells within the body and removes their waste products. Cells are the basic building blocks of life – varying in size, shape and function. Groups of cells form body tissues, such as skin and muscle, or make up organs, such as the brain and heart. Cells require a constant supply of oxygen and nutrients to produce the energy needed to fuel the thousands of different chemical activities within the body. During the process of creating energy, known as cell metabolism, various waste products, such as carbon dioxide and water, are released into the spaces between the cells. If the blood circulation is poor, the cells are starved of oxygen and nutrients, and toxins begin to accumulate in the tissues.

The healthy circulation of blood is essential to the health and vitality of all the bodily systems. When the blood circulation to the cells is sluggish or impaired, energy levels plummet, muscles may feel stiff, painful and tired, the brain starts to suffer lapses in concentration and memory, hair looks lacklustre, skin takes on a dull appearance and spots may develop. Indian head massage can boost the flow of blood through the cells in the brain, scalp, face, neck and shoulders, helping to keep the mind alert and the body active and promoting fresh, clear skin and healthy, vibrant hair.

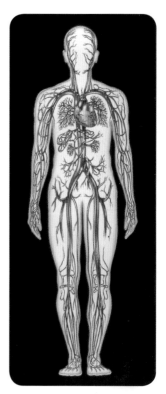

The organs and blood vessels of the human body that work together to enable the circulation of blood.

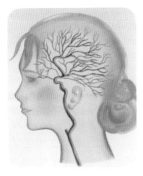

The red (oxygenated) and blue (deoxygenated) blood to and from the head.

Continuous circuit

Blood is pumped around the body by the heart, a hollow muscular bag that forces the blood through a continuous figure-of-eight circuit, travelling between the lungs, the heart and the tissues of the body. It carries unwanted carbon dioxide from the cells to the lungs to be exhaled and then collects the freshly inhaled oxygen and distributes it around the body. Blood picks up nutrients, such as glucose, vitamins and minerals, from the digestive tract and delivers this nourishment to the cells. Toxic waste products are dropped off at the lungs and sweat glands to be eliminated, or taken to the liver where they are prepared for excretion by the kidneys. Blood also carries heat around the body and takes hormones from the endocrine glands, where they are produced, to the target organs, where they trigger a reaction.

Transporting supplies

Blood that is rich in fresh oxygen is known as oxygenated blood. This oxygen-rich blood surges from the heart under pressure into a network of blood vessels called arteries. Blood is travelling under such pressure that if you cut an artery it would bleed profusely. When the heart contracts and pumps out blood, the thick, elastic walls of the arteries expand slightly and then return to their normal shape as the heart relaxes. The wave of pressure that causes this temporary change in shape in the artery wall is felt as the pulse.

✦ Press very gently on the carotid artery at the side of your neck and you will feel your pulse. If you have difficulty locating it, trace a line down from your earlobe to the hollow under your jaw. The number of pulses that occur in a minute is known as the pulse rate. This is the same as the number of times the heart beats in a minute. The normal pulse rate for an adult at rest varies between 60

and 80 beats a minute. This increases with activity, stress and strong emotions.

Blood pressure

When the heart contracts, blood is pumped into the arteries. When it relaxes, blood flows into the heart from the veins. The force with which the heart pumps blood through the arteries is known as blood pressure. This is usually based on two measurements. The force exerted when the heart contracts is known as the systolic blood pressure; the reduction in force when the heart relaxes is known as diastolic pressure. Blood pressure often changes, rising with exercise and strong emotions such as stress, for example. Fluctuations in blood pressure are normal but a permanently raised level can be detrimental to health and is a contributory factor in strokes and heart disease.

If the blood was not under pressure it would naturally gravitate to the lower parts of the body. Blood pressure ensures that some blood is forced upward through the aorta, the largest artery in the body. The aorta branches into the carotid arteries on either side of the neck, which divide and sub-divide into smaller arteries to supply the tissues of the brain, face and scalp. Most arteries lie deep within the body, where they are protected by muscles and bones, but the carotid arteries are near the surface of the neck. When massaging this area, it is important not to press too heavily as you could interrupt the flow of blood to the brain, possibly causing unconsciousness.

Fair exchange

Arteries continually branch into smaller and smaller arteries until they become tiny arterioles, which divide into a network of blood capillaries. Capillaries are only one cell thick, which allows blood plasma (the liquid base of blood, holding nutrients and other substances in solution) to seep through the thin capillary walls, where it becomes known as tissue fluid. This fluid acts as a medium for the exchange of nourishing oxygen and nutrients with the unwanted carbon dioxide and waste products. The cells absorb the nourishment from the tissue fluid and, at the same time, eliminate their waste products through diffusion into the tissue fluid and then through the thin capillary walls back into the bloodstream.

Deoxygenated blood, which contains very little oxygen, is carried back to the heart via the venous (vein) system. These blood vessels begin as tiny venules that gradually increase in size to become a network of veins. This blood is under much less pressure than blood in the arterial system and so many veins have non-return valves to prevent a back-flow of blood. In general, veins are closer to the surface of the skin than arteries. Blood drains from the head, largely by the force of gravity, via the jugular veins, which join the two main veins – the superior and inferior vena cava – leading directly to the heart. Once the deoxygenated blood arrives back at the heart, it is ready to begin its journey to the lungs and around the body again.

Monitoring the flow

The amount of oxygenated blood delivered to the cells is determined by the arterioles. The walls of these tiny blood vessels can expand and contract considerably to control their output and ensure that cells are supplied with exactly the right quantity of blood for their needs. If any area needs extra energy, such as the muscles when exercising, oxygenated blood is diverted from other parts of the body to satisfy the demand. This is known as blood shunting. As the blood vessels in the working area dilate to allow extra blood to enter, there is a reddening, known as erythema, that gives the skin a radiant glow.

Heat transfer

Blood also carries heat, so the increased flow through the cells will automatically warm the tissues. The production of energy in the cells generates a huge amount of heat. This is carried in the blood where it is evenly distributed around the body to maintain a constant temperature of around 37°C (98.6°F). If too much heat is produced, the "superficial" blood vessels – near the surface of the skin – dilate so that excess heat can be carried to the surface and dissipated into the atmosphere. If the temperature outside the body is cold, the superficial blood vessels constrict to conserve heat and the skin takes on a more sallow appearance.

Blood composition

Blood contains 55 per cent plasma and 45 per cent blood cells, such as erythrocytes, leucocytes and platelets.

- Plasma is a straw-coloured liquid. It is 91 per cent water and holds sugar, amino acids, mineral salts, enzymes and other substances in solution.
- Erythrocytes, or red blood cells, contain haemoglobin, a protein that absorbs oxygen from the lungs and releases it to the body cells. The erythrocytes appear dark red when haemoglobin is carrying oxygen, but the colour changes to a paler red once the oxygen has been released.
- Leucocytes, or white blood cells, play a vital part in the immune system by attacking and destroying infectious micro-organisms, such as bacteria, and producing antibodies to guard against future infection.

- Platelets, or thrombocytes, are capable of sticking together to form a clot or mass, especially when blood is exposed to the air, as a result of a cut, for example. This binding action seals the wound to prevent bleeding, fluid loss and infection.

It is important to remember that Indian head massage is designed to complement – and not replace – orthodox medical treatment. Therefore, it should not be seen as an alternative to your own doctor's diagnosis and treatment.

CHECKLIST

Indian head massage and blood circulation

- Indian head massage works with the circulatory system.

- The various massage manipulations can help improve the flow of deoxygenated blood back to the heart and speed the flow of freshly oxygenated blood to the superficial and deeper tissues of the neck, shoulders and head.

- A more efficient flow of arterial blood enables more oxygen and nutrients to be brought to the cells, so aiding their proper functioning and stimulating cell growth, division, renewal and healing.

- A speedier flow of venous blood back to the heart helps remove carbon dioxide and metabolic waste products at a quicker rate. This helps muscles function more efficiently, prevents muscle stiffness and pain and improves the condition of hair and skin.

- The increased supply of blood produces warmth, which promotes general relaxation (the same effect as lying in a warm bath) and encourages small amounts of oil to be absorbed through the skin.

- Massage causes dilation of the superficial blood vessels, which gives a healthy glow to the skin. The generally relaxing effect of massage can help to lower a permanently raised blood pressure.

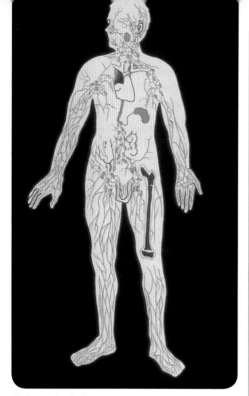

The human lymphatic system.

⊛ Lymphatic system

We are bombarded by toxins that can enter the body in many ways – including through food and drink, pollution in the air and the invasion of bacteria and viruses. Toxic waste matter is also created internally as a by-product of normal metabolic processes. The body has a highly efficient self-cleansing system to eliminate these potentially harmful substances from the body through the skin, the kidneys, the colon, the immune system and the lymphatic system. When these systems slow down, toxins are able to accumulate and circulate around the body. This can give rise to a number of symptoms, including tiredness, nasal and sinus conges-tion, susceptibility to coughs and colds, frequent headaches, puffiness, disturbed sleep and dull skin and hair.

Indian head massage can help discourage the build up of toxic matter in the head, neck and shoulders by boosting the efficiency of the lymphatic system. This system is an intricate network of glands, vessels and tubes that extends through-out the body, removing viruses, bacteria and other foreign materials and draining excess fluid from tissue spaces. The

lymphatic system is integrally linked with the circulation of blood. However, it has several differences. It does not have a muscular pump equivalent to the heart and it does not form a complete circuit around the body. It is a one-way system of tubes that takes fluid from the body tissues to the heart but does not collect fluid from the heart.

The flow of lymph

The fluid that travels through the lymphatic system is known as lymph. This straw-coloured liquid is derived from the tissue fluid that bathes the body's cells. Tissue fluid contains both unwanted waste matter, which has been eliminated by the cells, and oxygen and nutrients, which have been delivered by the arterial bloodstream to nourish the cells. Once the cells have absorbed what they need for maintenance, growth and repair, most of the fluid and waste materials are returned to the bloodstream through the thin walls of the blood capillaries. The remaining fluid and foreign matter becomes lymph and seeps through the walls of the lymph capillaries to enter the lymphatic system.

Unlike blood capillaries, which have a venous and an arterial end, lymph vessels are blind-ended tubes. The walls of lymph vessels are more permeable than those of blood capillar-ies, allowing them to absorb larger particles of foreign material, cell debris, bacteria and viruses in the tissue fluid. They also drain any excess fluid that has built up as a result of infection, tissue damage or the presence of a foreign body. If drainage is sluggish, it can lead to puffiness, or water retention. Some nutrients pass through the vessel walls, but lymph contains fewer nutrients and less oxygen than blood. Lymph vessels in the small intestine absorb fat, which is slowly emptied into the bloodstream.

Lymph vessels join together to form a network of tubes that carry lymph to the heart. Lymph is forced through the vessels by the rhythmic relaxation and contraction of nearby muscles during breathing and other body movements. Regular exercise has been shown to have a beneficial impact on lymph drainage. To ensure the lymph travels in the right direction, some lym-phatic vessels have non-return valves that prevent back-flow. Lymphatic vessels get progressively larger until they eventually empty into two ducts: the right lymphatic duct and the thoracic duct. These two ducts drain the lymph into the subclavian veins at the base of the neck and finally into the vena cava, where it mixes with venous blood and is carried to the heart.

🐾 *The skin complements the lymphatic system by playing a major role in eliminating toxins from the body. These waste products are released in the sweat that seeps through the pores. A buildup of dirt, grime and dead skin cells can block the pores.*

Use a loofah or body brush regularly on your body as this helps purge the body of toxins by stimulating the lymphatic system and sloughing off dull, dead cells on the skin's surface.

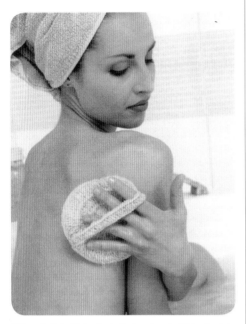

Aid your body in eliminating toxins by using a loofah to stimulate a sluggish lymphatic system.

Cleansing and defending

All lymphatic vessels drain through lymph nodes, or "glands", which are placed in strategic positions along the network. Lymph nodes are small, oval-shaped structures that act as filters to cleanse the lymph and remove any potentially harmful micro-organisms before they are allowed to enter the bloodstream and travel from one part of the body to another. Cancer cells may also be spread along the lymph vessels. There are around 100 lymph nodes in the body and these vary greatly in size – some are as small as the head of a pin while others are as large as an almond. They are grouped into clusters that can lie near the surface or deeper in the body and drain a particular area. Lymph passes through several lymph nodes on its journey to the heart.

Lymph nodes store two types of leucocyte, or white blood cell – phagocytes and lymphocytes – that are part of the cleansing and filtering process. Phagocytes trap, engulf and digest unwanted matter, such as dirt, dead cells and destroyed bacteria. Lymphocytes produce antibodies to combat viruses and bacteria. The lymphatic system also comprises organs such as the spleen, thymus gland and tonsils that play a major role in protecting and defending the body from infection and disease.

Whenever there is a threat of invasion by disease organisms, the lymph nodes in the area produce extra lymphocytes to repel the invaders. It is the accumulation of soldier cells and dead germs that causes the lymph nodes to become hard, swollen, inflamed and tender whenever the body is fighting a major disease. We have all experienced swollen lymph "glands" in our neck when suffering a throat infection. Disease organisms and white blood cells travel along the lymph vessels until they reach the nearest set of lymph nodes. An infected hand, for example, may result in swollen lymph nodes in the armpit. It is important not to massage over swollen lymph nodes as this may interfere with the body's natural defence procedures.

♪ Manual lymph drainage is a specific form of massage therapy that uses a gentle, pumping action to stimulate the lymphatic system and drain the buildup of fluids and toxins. Massage strokes are always performed in the direction of the lymphatic pathways – toward the heart.

☺ Muscles and bones

Indian head massage works on the many different muscles in the face, scalp, upper back, neck and shoulders. When these muscles are tense, the flow of blood and lymph through the tissues is restricted, leading to reduced supplies of fresh oxygen and nutrients and a buildup of stagnant wastes. This leads to stiffness, aches and pains, eye strain and feelings of anxiety and may contribute to greying and early hair loss. Massage helps relax tense muscles, thus stimulating the flow of blood and lymph through the area and easing tension headaches, aiding joint mobility, increasing concentration levels, encouraging healthy hair growth and promoting a general sense of well-being.

Muscle control

There are three different types of muscle within the body. Indian head massage is applied to the voluntary muscles, which, as the name implies, are the muscles over which we have conscious control to bring about movement – whether it is raising the shoulders or lowering the eyelids. Voluntary muscles are also known as skeletal muscles because they move and support the skeleton. Most of these muscles are attached to bones that pivot around joints. Different types of joints allow a varying range of movement. The bones of the skull, for example, are locked tightly together to form a protective casing for the brain and sense organs, whereas the shoulder joints are designed to allow for greater freedom of movement.

☀ There are around 650 voluntary muscles, which make up around 40–50 per cent of body weight. Some are large and powerful, allowing movements such as climbing and running; others help perform very accurate and precise movements.

Voluntary muscles are attached to the bones on either side of a joint by fibres of connective tissue, known as tendons. Muscles exert a pull on the tendon, which moves the bone and any weight it is carrying. This action enables an arm to be raised, for example, or the head to be turned. Muscles work in pairs. When one contracts to raise a bone, the other will relax to facilitate movement. You can see this process in action by moving your lower arm up and down. As your biceps muscle contracts to raise your lower arm, your triceps muscle relaxes – and vice versa.

Muscle fibres

Muscles are made up of a collection of many long cells, or fibres, which are enclosed in a tough sheet of connective tissue, known as a muscle sheath. Each fibre is made up of bundles of even thinner strands, called myofibrils. These myofibrils comprise even finer strands, called filaments. When a muscle contracts, the filaments slide over each other and the muscle becomes shorter and fatter. When a muscle relaxes, the filaments slide back and the muscle returns to its original length. Voluntary muscles are usually stimulated to contract or relax by messages sent from the brain to the motor nerve cells controlling the muscle fibres.

Muscles have their own supply of blood and lymphatic vessels. As the muscle relaxes, oxygenated blood flows in to nourish the tissues; as the muscle contracts, deoxygenated blood is forced out, carrying away waste products. The energy the muscles requires comes from oxygen, combined with its stores of a simple sugar called glycogen. This sets off a chemical process that releases both energy and heat. If supplies of oxygen are limited, or the muscles are working so vigorously that oxygen is used up quicker than the body can deliver it, a waste product, called lactic acid, is produced. This adversely affects the efficiency of the muscle, leading to muscle fatigue and pain, which usually passes quickly.

Muscular aches and pains

Some muscle fibres are always partially contracted, even while resting. This partial contraction, known as muscle tone, is essential for maintaining posture. Without muscle tone we would collapse under the force of gravity. Muscle tone also adds definition and shape to the body. However, if muscles are held in an abnormal state of contraction for long periods of time – for example, when sitting hunched over a steering wheel or computer screen, holding the telephone receiver between your chin and shoulder, or sleeping on a soft mattress – the normal contraction/relaxation sequence does not occur and the flow of blood and lymph through the fibres is impeded.

Under these adverse conditions, the muscle is slowly starved of oxygen and nutrients and toxic waste products begin to accumulate and stagnate, making the situation even worse. Over time, the muscle tissue gradually begins to change in structure. The connective tissue may start to thicken and fibres stick together so they can no longer slide over each other so easily. Some tense muscles can be felt as hard lumps or nodules beneath the skin, a condition known as fibrositis, which is often most apparent in the muscles of the shoulder and upper back. This situation means there is little space for the free flow of blood and lymph. Unfortunately, muscular tension tends to build up so slowly that we often do not realize what is happening until the sensory nerve receptors in the area register soreness, discomfort, aching and pain.

⊛ Bones of the head, neck and shoulders

It is important to have some idea of the position of the underlying structures so you know which areas to massage – and which to avoid. It is particularly important not to exert any pressure on the spine. This bony column protects the spinal cord and a vast number of individual nerves connecting the brain to the rest of the body.

Skull

The skull is at the top of the vertebral column. It is divided into two sets of bones forming the cranium and the face. The cranium is the part of the skull that surrounds and protects the brain. It consists of eight immovable bones. The following ones are of relevance to Indian head massage.

- One occipital bone forms the lower back of the cranium.
- Two parietal bones form the sides of the cranium and the roof of the head.
- Two temporal bones form the sides of the head around the ears.
- One frontal bone forms the forehead.

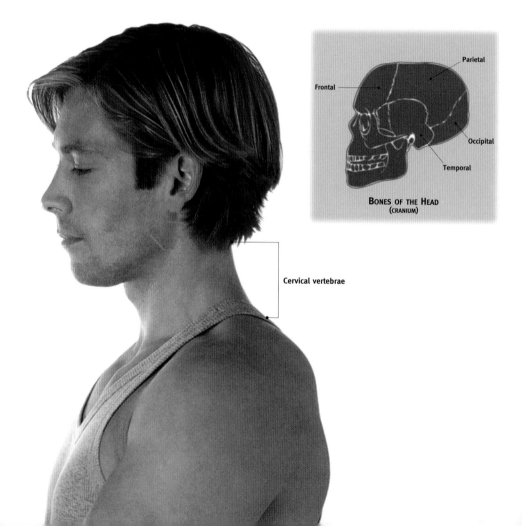

Frontal

Parietal

Occipital

Temporal

BONES OF THE HEAD
(CRANIUM)

Cervical vertebrae

Face

The face is formed from fourteen bones. The following ones are of particular relevance to Indian head massage.

- Two zygomatic bones form the cheekbones.
- Two maxilla bones form the upper jaw and hold the upper teeth.
- One mandible bone forms the lower jaw and holds the lower teeth. This is the largest and strongest of the facial bones.

Neck

The neck is made up of seven cervical vertebrae, which form the top of the spinal column and the neck.

- First vertebra supports the head.
- Second vertebra allows rotation of the head.

Shoulders

The shoulders are formed by the following bones.

- Two scapulas (shoulder blades). These triangular-shaped bones in the upper back are attached to muscles that move the arm.
- Two clavicles (collar-bones), one on either side of the sternum (breastbone). These long bones form a joint with the sternum and scapulas, allowing movement of the shoulders.

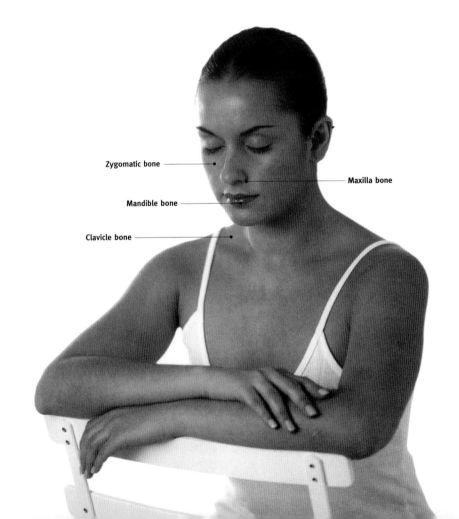

Zygomatic bone

Maxilla bone

Mandible bone

Clavicle bone

Muscles of the head, neck and shoulders

It is helpful to be able to locate the main muscles of the face, skull, neck, upper back and shoulders so you can be sure that you are massaging in the right place for optimum benefits.

Muscles of the neck, shoulders and upper back

The following muscles are responsible for controlling the head, neck and shoulder area.

- Two sterno-cleido mastoid muscles work together to bend the head. Individually, they allow rotation of the head sideways toward the shoulder.
- One trapezius muscle draws the shoulders together and downward, pulls the head backward and allows movement of the shoulder.
- Two deltoid muscles raise the arm sideways away from the side of the body and help draw it backward and forward.

Muscles for chewing

The following muscles are responsible for chewing (mastication).

- Masseter clenches the teeth and raises and closes the lower jaw tightly for chewing.
- Temporalis raises the lower jaw and presses it against the upper jaw to aid chewing.

Muscles of facial expression

The following muscles are mainly responsible for facial expression.

- Frontalis raises the eyebrows in surprise.
- Corrugator draws the eyebrows together in a frown.
- Orbicularis oculi closes the eyelid to wink.
- Risorius draws the corners of the mouth outward to grin.
- Buccinator compresses the cheeks to blow.
- Zygomaticus (major and minor) lifts the corners of the mouth upward and outward to smile.
- Orbicularis oris closes the mouth and purses the lips to kiss and whistle.
- Triangularis draws down the corners of the mouth to show sadness.
- Mentalis raises the lower lip, thereby wrinkling the chin, to indicate doubt.
- Platysma draws the corners of the mouth downward and backward to show horror.

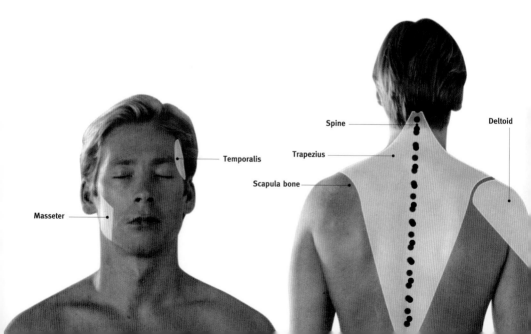

Masseter · Temporalis · Spine · Trapezius · Scapula bone · Deltoid

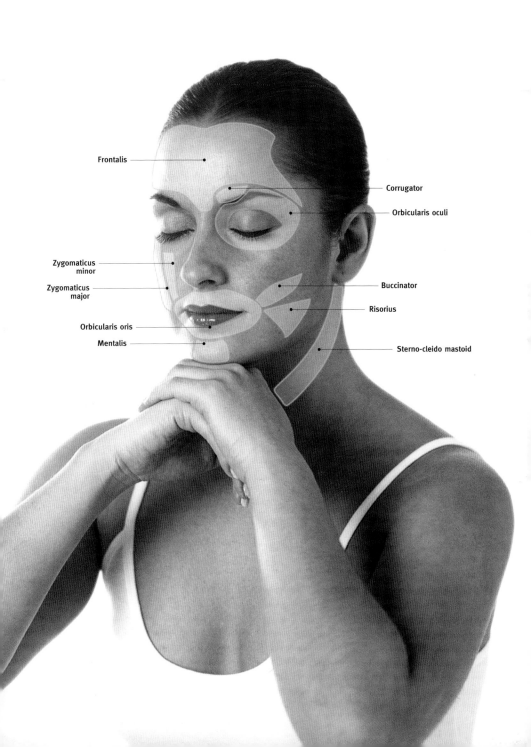

Frontalis

Corrugator

Orbicularis oculi

Zygomaticus
minor

Zygomaticus
major

Buccinator

Risorius

Orbicularis oris

Mentalis

Sterno-cleido mastoid

The average adult head weighs between three and four kilos, so the supporting muscles have to work very hard to co-ordinate its movements. The head is actually designed to balance on the upper neck vertebrae. However, most of us tend to push our heads forward when carrying out routine actions such as walking or watching television and this imposes an enormous strain on the muscles of the shoulders, back and neck. This tension tends to spread to the tissues that cover the skull, thereby impeding the flow of blood and lymph and leading to headaches, eye strain, stiffness and undernourished skin and hair roots.

Muscles of expression

Many of the muscles in the face are tiny and very delicate. They are attached to the facial skin so that when they contract, they literally "pull a face" – that is, they pull on the skin to create a facial expression. If these muscles become tense and taut through frowning, worry or pain they lose their flexibility and the face tends to look hard and set. It only takes 17 muscles to make you smile, but 43 for the average frown.

Indian head massage and muscle

The various massage techniques work on muscle tissue in different ways to help relax tense muscle fibres, tone slack fibres and increase blood and lymph flow through the tissues.

- The increased flow of oxygenated blood to the muscles brings fresh supplies of oxygen and nutrients to the muscle fibres.
- At the same time, a speedier venous flow and more efficient lymphatic drainage helps to prevent a buildup of waste products. This helps improve efficiency, aids repair and recovery and reduces pain, stiffness and muscle fatigue.
- The increased blood flow and frictional heat create warmth in the area. This encourages the muscles to relax so they are more receptive to the benefits of massage. The muscle fibres are stretched, broadened and separated, and any adhesions are broken down, enabling muscles to contract and relax more efficiently. The layer of tissue covering the skull is relaxed, which reduces headaches and eye strain and allows the hair follicles to be well supplied with nourishment, so encouraging healthy hair growth.
- Massage aids mobility of the neck and shoulder joints. Some facial muscles are encouraged to relax, which helps erase fine tension lines, while others are toned to give a younger, fresher appearance. Massage can also be an aid to greater awareness of the muscular tension that is being stored in the body by everyday activities.

⊛ Skin and hair

Massage with nourishing oils has long been used by Indian women as part of their beauty routine to promote strong, lustrous hair and keep their skin healthy, soft and supple. Scalp massage cannot reverse baldness or greying, which are often hereditary, but may help prevent excessive hair loss and will certainly make your hair soft, silky and shiny, with a natural bounce. Similarly, facial massage cannot remove wrinkles, which are largely due to smoking, pollution and excessive exposure to the damaging rays of the sun. However, by relaxing the underlying muscles, boosting the blood and lymph circulation and helping to shed dead skin cells, massage can give your face a younger, more attractive appearance.

The skin is one of nature's finest works of art. This complex organ, the largest in the body, provides a highly flexible protective covering to keep the body fluids in and to shield the internal structures and systems from injury and invasion by harmful micro-organisms. The skin contains thousands of sensory nerve endings that make it extremely sensitive to heat, cold, pain, light touch and deep pressure. The different sensory receptors respond to specific stimuli and send messages about these stimuli to the brain. The brain may respond by stimulating the motor nerves to carry out an appropriate action – such as tensing with pain or cold, or relaxing with the enjoyment of a pampering touch.

There is a large number of sensory nerve receptors in the face and scalp so massage to these areas can be particularly effective in influencing moods. Massage movements may be adapted to create a soothing and calming effect or to stimulate and invigorate. Appropriate selection of massage techniques for the face and scalp area can have a profound effect on the mind and body.

⊛ Skin structure

The skin has three main layers, the epidermis, the dermis, and the subcutaneous, or "below the skin", layer, each with a different composition and function.

Epidermis

The top skin layer is called the epidermis and is the one that can be seen and touched. It has no blood vessels and only a small number of nerve endings. This layer is where cell renewal takes place. The skin is made up of millions of cells that are constantly growing and replacing themselves. Over a period of around 27 days, cells push up through the epidermis, gradually changing in structure. Their nuclei (cell control centres) break down and the fluid within the cells is replaced by keratin, a tough and durable protein that makes the skin so hard-wearing. Skin cells have died by the time they reach the surface of the epidermis. As old cells are shed, fresh ones take their place and so the cycle continues. If these dead, scaly cells are allowed to accumulate, they give the skin a dull appearance.

◐ Dead skin cells are continually being rubbed off by the friction of everyday activities such as towel drying or wearing clothes that brush against the skin. It is estimated that around 80 per cent of household dust is made up of dead skin cells and that we shed a complete surface layer every five days.

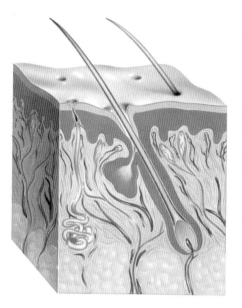

A cross-section of human skin. A hair pokes through the epidermis from the follicle or pit that holds it.

Some of the cells in the epidermis react with the sun's ultraviolet rays to produce a dark-brown pigment called melanin, which blocks some of the harmful effects of the sun. Melanin is mainly responsible for the normal colour of skin and hair – the more melanin there is, the darker the skin colour. Another function of the epidermis is to produce vitamin D – "the sunshine vitamin". When skin is exposed to the sun, its cells form vitamin D, which combines with calcium and phosphorus to develop and help maintain a healthy bone structure. A daily quota of sunlight is essential to health and well-being, but over-exposure can have a detrimental effect, not only on your health but also on your skin, leading to wrinkles, age-spots and a leathery appearance. This is why it is important to protect your skin during very sunny weather.

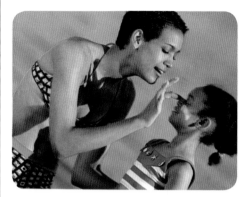

Protection from the sun, whether by using sunscreen or some form of shade, is important to protect our body's and face's delicate skin.

Dermis

The dermis lies directly underneath the epidermis and its main function is to support and nourish the epidermis. The dermis contains blood and lymph vessels, nerve endings, sweat and sebaceous glands and hair follicles. It is a much thicker layer than the epidermis and is made up of two types of protein fibres, collagen and elastin. Collagen strengthens the skin and protects against over-stretching. Elastin, as the name suggests, gives the skin its elasticity and allows it to regain its shape after it has been stretched – following pregnancy, for example. These fibres weaken and become stretched with age, so the skin tends to become looser and more wrinkled over time.

The dermis has tiny projections, known as papillae, that extend into the epidermis. Papillae contain nerve endings and blood and lymph vessels to ensure a healthy flow of blood and lymph around the living cells of the top layer. The blood vessels in the dermis also help maintain a constant internal body temperature of 37°C (98.6°F). If the body gets too hot, the blood vessels leading to the skin dilate to allow more warm blood to come to the surface so that the excess heat is lost. If the body gets too cold, the blood vessels near the skin constrict to stop too much heat from escaping.

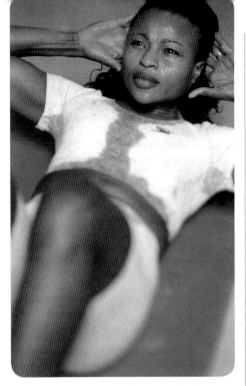

Exercise causes the body to sweat and so promote the elimination of toxins.

Removing heat and toxins

Sweating, or perspiration, is the body's other main reaction to raised temperature. The skin contains two to three million sweat glands, each consisting of a coiled section in the dermis, where sweat is produced, and a long tube that leads directly on to the surface of the skin through an opening called a pore. Sweat extracts heat from the blood flowing just beneath the surface and then oozes out through the pores. As the sweat evaporates, it removes heat from the skin. Some sweat glands respond to factors such as heat and exercise, others to emotional and hormonal changes. The sweat glands also play a major part in the body's excretory system and help eliminate toxic waste products through the pores. It is important to wash and rinse your skin thoroughly to prevent debris blocking the pores and hindering the flow of toxins from the body.

◆ The skin is used as a diagnostic tool in traditional Eastern medicine, as the colour and texture can indicate areas of ill-health within the body. As general health and well-being increases with regular Indian head massage, so the condition of the skin and hair will also improve.

Natural moisturizer

The dermis contains sebaceous glands, which secrete an oily liquid known as sebum. Sebum is a natural moisturizer, helping to keep the skin and hair soft and supple. Sebaceous glands tend to be more active following puberty, which accounts for the oiliness of the skin and hair during adolescence. When these glands are underactive, skin and hair tend to be very dry. Sebum helps keep the skin waterproof and combines with sweat to create an acidic coating, known as the acid mantle, to guard against the growth of bacteria and fungi. Harsh soaps and chemicals can upset the balance of this natural coating, so a mild cleanser suitable for your skin type is recommended.

◆ Skin varies in thickness over the body. The thinnest part is around the eyes, where it is only 0.5mm thick. The thickest part is on the palms and soles of the feet, where it is around 6mm thick.

Subcutaneous layer

The subcutaneous layer lies beneath the dermis and contains connective tissue, known as adipose tissue, where fat is stored. The subcutaneous layer helps to conserve body heat. Fat is a poor conductor of heat, thereby reducing heat loss through the skin. It also acts as a protective cushion for the bones and underlying internal organs.

Hair growth

Hair grows up through hollow spaces in the dermis known as hair follicles. Hair follicles are found all over the body except on the palms of the hands, soles of the feet, lips and the nipples. At the bottom of each hair follicle is an area known as the hair papilla where the living, growing cells are nourished and drained of toxins by the blood and lymph vessels in the dermis. Stress and illness can affect healthy hair growth. This is because the body does not regard hair as being essential to life, so in times of crisis blood may be diverted away from the cells in the hair follicles toward more important areas that are in need of extra oxygen and nutrients. If the living cells continue to be deprived of essential nourishment, scalp problems may develop and the hair roots can start to weaken, leading to dull, brittle hair and even mild hair loss.

Cells in the hair papilla multiply to form the hair root and shape the hair bulb and then push up through the follicle in the same way that skin cells migrate up through the epidermis. As the cells move upward through the follicle, they change their structure, fill with the durable protein keratin and eventually die. There are around 120,000 hairs on the average head. Each hair grows at a rate of around 1mm every three to four days. Over a period of between one and six years, an individual hair fibre grows, then stops, rests, degenerates and falls out. Around 50–100 hairs are lost from the head each day. Before a hair is shed, there is usually another one ready to replace it. If hairs are not replaced then patches of baldness occur.

The visible strands of hair are all dead tissue. Each strand has an inner shaft, containing a pigment that gives the hair its colour, and an outer cuticle. The cuticle protects the interior of the hair shaft and is lubricated by sebum, the body's natural moisturizer, secreted from sebaceous glands at the base of the hair root. Sebum makes the hair soft to touch and reflects light to give a glossy sheen. If the cuticle is damaged by too vigorous brushing, chemical treatments or excessive exposure to the sun, the hair can become coarse and prone to tangling.

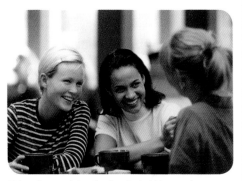

Hair varies not only in colour but also in thickness and type, resulting in straight or curly locks.

🐾 *The shape and size of the hair follicle determines the thickness and type of hair. Follicles with round openings produce straight hair, while follicles with oval openings produce curly or wavy hair.*

There are thousands of hair follicles in the dermis, each one attached to a small muscle called an arrector pili, which is activated by a motor nerve. When a person feels cold or has a sudden fright, these muscles respond by making the strand of hair stand on end. Small bumps are formed over the skin, giving the appearance of a plucked goose – hence the term "goose bumps".

🐾 *Traditional treatments for preventing baldness include rubbing a fresh cut onion on the scalp or applying stinging nettles to stimulate the blood circulation. An Indian head massage is a far more pleasant treatment!*

Indian head massage and skin and hair

Massage has many beneficial effects on the condition of the skin and hair.

- The circulation of blood and lymph is stimulated, thereby delivering fresh supplies of nutrients and oxygen to the living cells and removing unwanted metabolic wastes and excess tissue fluid. This provides a healthy environment for cell growth, renewal, repair and division.
- Massage also aids desquamation, or the shedding of dead skin cells, as it stimulates cell division, so more cells move up toward the surface. The friction of the hands also helps to rub off dead cells. Fresh new cells are exposed, which improves the appearance and texture of the skin.
- Massage leads to dilation of superficial blood capillaries, which gives a healthy glow to a sallow complexion. The sebaceous glands are stimulated to produce more sebum, which keeps the skin and hair soft and supple, and raises the temperature of the skin, which ensures optimum benefits from any oils used.
- Massage also has a cleansing effect by stimulating the sweat glands to produce more sweat, which assists the removal of metabolic wastes and helps prevent the pores getting clogged with dirt and dead skin cells.

⊛ Stress factor

Stress affects us all, whether adults or children, from the first jangle of the alarm clock in the morning to the final struggle with the duvet cover at night. It is the natural response to any kind of extra demand, pressure or change, pleasant or unpleasant, placed on the mind or body. Stress is often given a bad name, but without it we would soon become bored and lethargic. It can provide the motivation to finish tasks, give a competitive edge when playing sport and raise performance at meetings and in exams. Stress provides the tingle before an exciting event and the exhilaration of a high-risk leisure activity. It can increase your self-confidence and boost your energy.

Stress is only harmful when the extra burden becomes too great to handle and you lose your ability to cope in a calm and rational way. It is a very personal response. Perhaps other factors become involved, the demands get too severe or go on for too long, circumstances change for the worse, or your support network breaks down. We all have different stress thresholds and these can vary under different circumstances. What is invigorating for one person at a certain time may cause anxiety in another situation. And we all respond to stress in different ways.

While some people react to even minor upsets by becoming aggressive and blaming everyone around them, others retreat into themselves. "I can't cope" and "It's all too much for me" are common cries when suffering from too many pressures in our lives.

Negative factors

Among the main causes of negative stress are major life crises or changes such as bereavement, divorce, moving house and starting a new job. In our fast-moving modern society, however, there are a very great number of potentially stressful situations – major or minor, at work and at home – that can build up over time and lead to mental, physical and emotional overload. The pressures may be external, such as a hostile boss, critical spouse, argumentative children, or even a constantly ringing telephone or the noise of road works in the street. They can also be internal, such as persistent worries about being made redundant, feelings of inadequacy or guilt about a relationship or event.

Physical tension and illness are also directly linked with mental and emotional health and well-being and can exacerbate the problem. We all know that when we are emotionally stressed or worried, our bodies respond with physical symptoms, and vice versa. Think how often anxieties about a family argument or a visit to the dentist have been transformed into a headache or stomach cramps, so making the situation even worse. When we are suffering from a headache or flu, we feel irritable and depressed, which, in turn, hinders our recovery. Our language is rich in sayings that reinforce the connection. We "grit our teeth" and "carry the weight of the world on our shoulders" and we complain that people "get under our skin" or "make us sick".

Fight or flight

When you are faced with a stressful situation, whether real or perceived, physical, mental or emotional, internal "alarm bells" sound and the body responds by secreting hormones such as adrenaline and cortisol to prepare for instant action. This "fight or flight" response is a primitive survival tactic to cope with a purely physical threat, such as an attack from a wild animal. Muscles contract for optimum performance, either in facing the attacker or making an instant getaway. The heart and lungs work extra hard to speed up the flow of blood and oxygen to the muscles and brain. Blood pressure and pulse rate rise. Breathing becomes quicker. Sugars and fats are released into the bloodstream. Blood is diverted from the skin

(causing it to go white) and the stomach (leading to the sensation of "butterflies") to provide the muscles and brain with extra supplies of energy. Hairs stand on end as protection against the attacker and to produce a more menacing look. Sweat glands produce more sweat to cool the body ready for the expected physical effort.

The fight or flight response was designed to prepare the body for rapid and efficient physical action in a crisis. In primitive days, normal functions were restored as soon as the threat was over and physical action, whether in fight or flight, had utilized the increased energy supplies circulating in the body. In modern times, however, although our stress is more often psychological, the body responds in the same way. As we have no physical outlet (except exercise which is very beneficial, or perhaps punching a pillow!), stress hormones build up and we live under a low level of "threat" for days, months and even years.

Stress levels are exacerbated by the constant demands made on you every day.

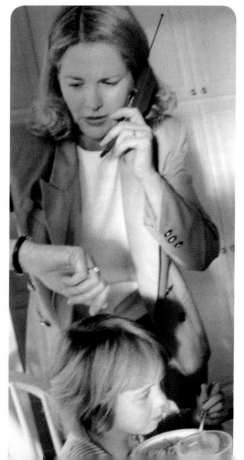

Effects of chronic stress

While short bursts of positive stress can be revitalizing, prolonged (chronic) negative stress keeps the mind and body in a constant state of mild "overdrive" and saps mental and physical energy. These effects often creep up so slowly that many people do not notice the changes within themselves. All aspects of life can be affected. Minor hassles become major traumas and you may find yourself lying awake at night with your mind buzzing. You may find it hard to concentrate at work and doubt your ability, so your productivity can decline. You may then swing between bouts of weeping, with feelings of helplessness and hopelessness, to fits of aggression, when you pick fights with colleagues and neighbours. You may feel so down that you cannot face getting out of bed in the morning or find yourself turning to food or alcohol to lift your mood. You may start to get unexplained stomach upsets, headaches and feel a stiffness in your neck and shoulder muscles.

When the body is exposed to excessive stress for long periods of time, physical and mental health can become seriously affected, largely because the stress hormones interfere with the circulatory and immune systems. If allowed to continue, chronic stress can lead to permanently raised blood pressure, digestive disorders, migraine, back pain, heart disease and skin and hair complaints. Stress hormones also depress the immune system, leading to greater susceptibility to diseases and allergies. Around 70 per cent of all illness is believed to be directly associated with physical, mental and emotional stress.

Indian head massage and stress

Indian head massage works simultaneously on a physical and psychological level, counteracting physical and mental tension or lethargy and encouraging well-being.

- On a physical level, massage relaxes tense and tight muscles, eases aches and pains, mobilizes the joints and regulates blood and lymph circulation, so restoring normal functioning. As the physical aches and pains are rubbed away, you will start to feel calmer and more able to cope with daily pressures in a relaxed and positive frame of mind.
- The deep physical and mental relaxation induced by massage has been proved effective in relieving the symptoms of stress, thus preventing serious health problems.
- On a psychological level, a massage gives you time to unwind so that nagging worries and problems can be viewed in a new light. The peace and quiet of massage allows the mind the time to relax and recharge. The caring, physical contact of massage helps boost self-esteem and encourages the release of "feel good" endorphins, which counteract the stress hormones in the bloodstream and boost the immune system, so helping to fight infection.
- Massage can facilitate the release of suppressed tension, which often brings a great sense of emotional relief. The relaxation effect encourages deep breathing, which relaxes the body and calms the mind.
- Massage can encourage an increased sense of self-awareness, which often leads to early recognition of stress signals and the realization of the need for mental and physical relaxation in everyday life.

CASE STUDY

Time for myself

On her 40th birthday, Janice, a full-time mother of four young children, was given a gift voucher for an Indian head massage. "I was really touched," she said. "It was such a thoughtful present, especially as it came with an offer to look after my children too, so there were no excuses. My friends are always telling me that I get so bogged down with the children and house that I rarely spend any time or money on myself. This is true, but I feel so guilty when I do. However, I thought that this was something that I would really enjoy. It doesn't involve too much time or needing to show off all your lumps and bumps.

"I was converted after the first five minutes. It was just heaven. I really look forward to my weekly sessions – and notice if I have to miss for some reason. It is my time, my indulgence, my pleasure. No constant demands, no responsibilities, no expectations, no telephone – just peace and quiet. My therapist always makes me feel really well looked after. My weekly 'time out' has helped me to see things in a different way. I have stopped worrying about little things – and now enjoy life more. I'm much less of a nag with my husband and children."

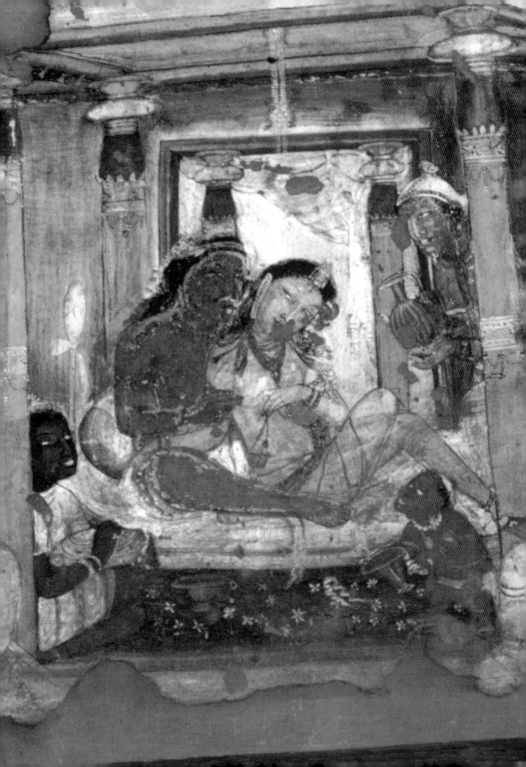

CHAPTER THREE

OILS FOR HEALTH AND BEAUTY

S INCE THE EARLIEST CIVILIZATIONS, plants and plant extracts have been valued for their medicinal and cosmetic qualities. Ancient healing systems, such as Ayurveda, recognized the power of plants to promote health and well-being, and the earliest cave drawings confirm that primitive dwellers used natural colours to paint and dye their hair. Over thousands of years, it was discovered that the nuts and seeds of plants also yielded oils that provide the ideal lubricating medium for massage and can be combined with pure essential oils to have specific health-giving effects on mind and body. The long tradition of using natural vegetable oils to enhance the benefits of massage continues to the present day.

Sixth Century Gupta cave painting of a scene in the Palace of Jataka, found in Ajanta, India.

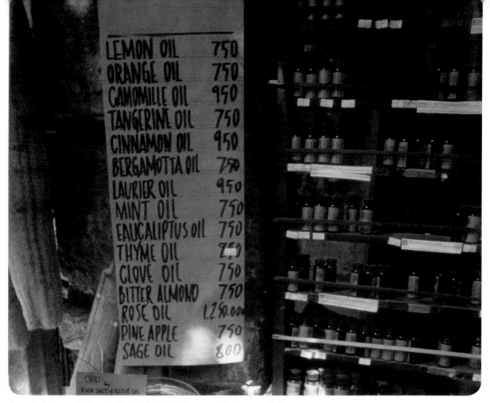

A wonderful array of oils can be found in health food stores and Indian grocer's shops.

۞ Why use oils?

Warm vegetable oils, often mixed with aromatic herbs and spices, are an essential part of a massage in India. These oils, which have become known as "carrier" oils in the West, act as a lubricant to make the massage a smoother and more pleasant experience for the giver and recipient. They also complement the circulation-boosting effects of head massage by cleansing the scalp and nourishing, moisturizing and strengthening the skin and hair. In the West, many people shy away from being seen in public with greasy-looking hair but in India it is very common for men, women and children to go about their daily lives with an oil-drenched head. Indeed, it is this tradition of regular head massage with vegetable carrier oils that helps protect their hair from the drying effect of the harsh sun and accounts for the beautifully lustrous locks so prized in Indian society.

۞ Choosing vegetable carrier oils

The main vegetable carrier oils used in Indian head massage are almond, coconut, mustard, olive, sesame and sunflower. You can obtain a selection of natural vegetable carrier oils from many health food stores, Indian grocer's shops, aromatherapy mail order suppliers and some supermarkets – but do choose the highest quality products. Check with a shop assistant before you buy, or ask a qualified aromatherapist to recommend some reputable suppliers. Look for oils that are unrefined, extracted mechanically by cold or warm pressing and free from additives. Most vegetable carrier oils sold for cooking are highly refined and are extracted using extremely high temperatures, which destroys much of the nutritional content. Although these oils will not cause any harm, they will not offer the same benefits either and you may well end up smelling like a wok or frying pan! If possible, select organic oils, as these have been produced without the use of chemical fertilizers or pesticides. Choose these more nutritious oils for dressing salads, too.

🌢 *If you or your massage partner have an allergy to nuts, avoid using nut oils as small quantities may be absorbed into the bloodstream.*

Oriental blends

There is a wide selection of ready blended scalp and hair oils, available in chemist's shops and department stores, that are suitable for Indian head massage. These blends are often formulated for different hair and skin types or mixed with herbs and essential oils to aid relaxation, increase energy levels or add an erotic note to the occasion. For an authentic touch, it is worth shopping around for blended oils imported directly from India and sold in Indian supermarkets and health stores. These oils are often blended with Eastern herbs, spices and fruits, such as brahmi and neem, which are not readily available in the West. Brahmi is a herb that is widely used in Ayurvedic medicine to balance all three doshas, stimulate the circulatory system and promote hair growth. Neem oil is extracted from the seeds of the neem tree, which is native to India and has cleansing and insecticide properties.

Commercial blended oils can provide a good starting point for using oils in head massage. They do vary greatly in texture and quality, however, so buy in small quantities and test a selection to identify the ones you prefer and find most enjoyable to use. Choose an oil that has a pleasant aroma and feels smooth on your hands. Some oils may have a rather unpleasant, synthetic aroma; others may leave a sticky residue on your hands and on the skin of your massage partner, or may be too watery to slide easily over the skin.

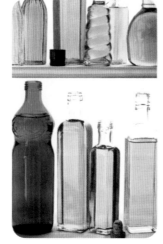

Take care when storing essential and blending oils.

✆ Pure essential oils

The vegetable oils used in Indian head massage can be applied on their own, mixed with another vegetable oil or blended with an appropriate pure essential oil. Pure essential oils are quite different from vegetable oils – and it is important not to confuse the two. Essential oils are non-greasy and extremely concentrated essences extracted from the petals, leaves, fruits and bark of aromatic plants. When used safely and correctly they can have a therapeutic effect on the mind, body and emotions. The oils enter the bloodstream in two ways: inhalation via the lungs and absorption through the skin.

Essential oils each have their own distinctive aromas that can have a profound influence on moods. The nasal passages contain large numbers of olfactory nerve receptors. These are closely linked to the part of the brain associated with emotions, arousal, feelings and memories. Certain smells can calm you down, wake you up or help you to concentrate. When blended with a vegetable carrier oil, tiny molecules of pure essential oils are absorbed through the skin and transported around the body to fulfil specific healing functions.

Choosing essential oils

A pure essential oil can enter the body within twenty minutes and may stay in the bloodstream for over 24 hours, so the purity of the product is crucial. Look for oils sold in dark glass bottles with a screw cap. They should be labelled "essential oil", which ensures that they contain 100 per cent concentrated plant oil. A good guide is to check that the labels show the common name as well as the botanical Latin name and have specific instructions for use, including safety guidelines. Look for a batch number and expiry date. Essential oils are sold in health food stores, chemist's shops and through mail-order outlets. They should be stored in a cabinet in a cool dark room and not on a shelf, where they may be exposed to light and heat. A qualified aromatherapist will be able to suggest a suitable supplier.

Blending oils

Pure essential oils should be treated with great respect. They are highly potent and can be toxic if misused. Do not make the mistake of thinking that the more oil you apply, the greater the benefits. This is not the case, so use only tiny quantities. Adding that extra drop could cause skin irritation and other harmful reactions. Initially, it is best to err

Using essential oils safely

The essential oils recommended on the following pages are safe for use in Indian head massage at home. However, you should always remember that all essential oils are very powerful and should be treated with caution.

- Never apply to the skin neat – always dilute with a carrier oil first. Wash off any spills immediately.

- Do not take internally.

- Keep bottles out of reach of children and pets.

- Avoid using any pure essential oils during pregnancy, when breastfeeding or on babies, children, or elderly people unless you are a fully qualified aromatherapist. Do not use in epilepsy, high blood pressure, asthma, hay fever or other allergic conditions, or any other contraindications (see page 65).

- Seek professional advice if you are taking homeopathic medicines, as some essential oils may adversely affect the treatment.

- Keep oils away from eyes. In case of accident, wash with plenty of water and seek medical advice.

- Do not use perfume or diffuse essential oils into the atmosphere while using essential oils for massage.

- Always obtain oils from a reputable source, make sure they are clearly labelled and always follow the instructions.

Before using essential oils, it is advisable to perform a skin test to check for sensitivity. Make up your chosen blend of oils. Rub a little of the blended oil on the inside of the wrist or behind the ears. Leave uncovered for 24 hours. Do not wash this area. Reactions often occur within a few hours. If you notice any signs of a rash, reddening or itchiness then you should not use the oil. Rinse off immediately with cold water.

on the side of caution and use just one drop of a single pure essential oil for every 10ml (two teaspoons) of vegetable carrier oil. In the case of some oils such as rose, jasmine and Roman chamomile, you should add one drop to 30ml (six teaspoons). As you gain knowledge and experience of using pure essential oils, you can experiment by using a wider selection and different quantities, or mixing oils to give a synergistic (multiple) effect – but always follow the instructions and adhere strictly to the safety precautions.

When blending oils, ensure that your hands and all utensils are clean and dry. Measure the required amount of carrier oil (10ml or 30ml) into a small bowl or a measuring bottle. It may be advisable to use a 5ml medicine spoon to ensure you use the right amount, as the size of teaspoons can vary enormously. Now add one drop of your chosen pure essential oil to the carrier oil – always buy essential oils in bottles with a special nozzle that allows you to measure one drop at a time accurately. Mix the oils in the bowl or shake the bottle, if it has a stopper. If you accidentally add more than one drop of essential oil, mix in the appropriate amount of extra carrier oil to restore the balance. Remember, essential oils are very concentrated. Wash your hands after blending.

Storing oils

Most kinds of carrier oil last for about six months before going rancid and becoming unsuitable for massage. Once blended with a pure essential oil, they should be used within a month. Keep your carrier and essential oils in dark glass bottles with screw lids and store in a cool place, out of direct sunlight. Undiluted essential oils should be kept in a locked medicine cupboard. Keep the lid firmly closed, as essential oils evaporate when exposed to the air. Most essential oils last from six months to a year, depending on the oil and how often it is used. Some essential oils, such as sandalwood and patchouli, have a much longer shelf-life and may even improve with age.

Essential and carrier oils should be kept in dark bottles.

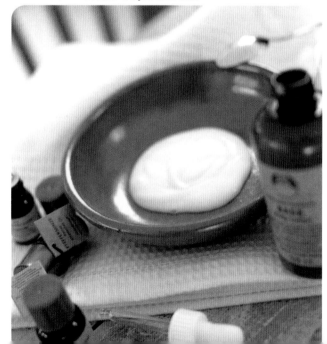

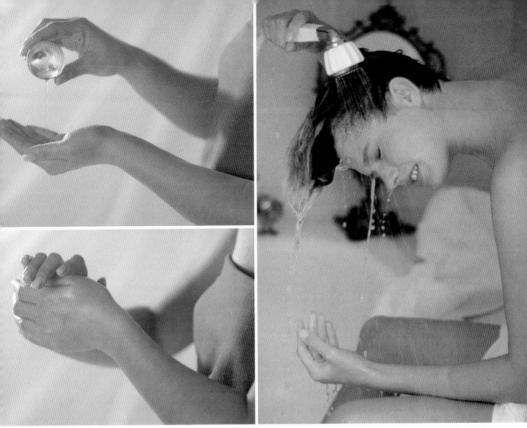

When removing oil after a head massage use shampoo first before rinsing.

☺ Applying oil

It is best to use around 10ml (two teaspoons) of oil for a head and shoulder massage. This may seem like a generous quantity but the hair does tend to absorb a lot of oil. The amount of oil you use will depend on your massage partner's hair length, skin texture and preference – and this can be adjusted on subsequent occasions. You need enough oil to allow your hands to "slip" over the skin in a smooth and comfortable way and to prevent the hair roots being unduly stressed by the massage, but not so much that your hands slide and you are unable to feel the underlying tissues.

Pour the oil into a small plastic bowl or plastic bottle. Glass is best avoided as it can easily slip through greasy hands. Place the container on a paper towel on a nearby surface. If you are using a bottle, choose one with an easy-to-use dispenser so that you can replenish the oil without interrupting the massage. With a small bowl, you can easily dip in one or two fingers if you need more lubrication.

If there is any oil left in the bowl at the end of the massage, throw it away immediately. Do not use it again, as it might spread infection if re-used.

Oil is best applied warm, as this provides a far more pleasant sensation for your partner and also encourages absorption of the natural healing chemicals in the oils to have a beneficial effect on mind and body. Skin temperature, or a little warmer, is ideal. Warm the blended oil by placing the receptacle near a radiator or pour some oil into one hand and rub your hands together briskly.

When washing out oil from your hair, put a small amount of shampoo directly on to your hair. The shampoo emulsifies the oil and can then be rinsed off more easily with warm water. Do not wet your hair first as the water will prevent the oil from combining with the shampoo and even after several washes, a film of oil will remain on the hair.

✍ Oils for hair types

Different types of hair have their own unique properties – and often problems – and so, when planning to give an Indian head massage, for the best results choose the most appropriate carrier and essential oils.

Normal hair

Normal hair is glossy and strong with plenty of body and bounce. It is an indication of good health and well-being.

CARRIER OILS TO CHOOSE ⤜ coconut, jojoba, sunflower.
ESSENTIAL OILS TO CHOOSE ⤜ lavender, patchouli, rose, rosemary.

Dry hair

This type of hair tends to be coarse, brittle and lacklustre. It tangles easily and may be fly-away and hard to control. Dryness is often caused by over-exposure to the dehydrating rays of the sun, or the use of strong shampoos, heated hair appliances, chemical treatments and colourants.

CARRIER OILS TO CHOOSE ⤜ coconut, jojoba, olive, sunflower, sweet almond.
ESSENTIAL OILS TO CHOOSE ⤜ frankincense, jasmine, rose, sandalwood.

Greasy hair

Greasy hair tends to be rather dull and lank. It sticks to the scalp and is difficult to style. Oiliness tends to be due to a fatty diet, stress or hormonal changes, which can lead to over-active sebaceous glands (oil glands in the skin). Oily hair is common during puberty and around menstruation.

CARRIER OILS TO CHOOSE ⤜ jojoba, sesame, sweet almond.
ESSENTIAL OILS TO CHOOSE ⤜ geranium, lavender, rosemary, sandalwood.

Dandruff

A common scalp complaint – dandruff is often itchy and can be embarrassing, but it is not contagious. Dandruff is thought to be due to an excessive buildup of dead skin cells that are not removed by washing. The underlying cause has not been positively identified, but stress, fatigue, cold weather and a poor diet can all play a part.

There are two types – dry and oily. Dry dandruff is characterized by dry, white flakes; oily dandruff by yellow, sticky flakes.

CARRIER OILS TO CHOOSE ⤜ coconut, sweet almond.
ESSENTIAL OILS TO CHOOSE ⤜ geranium, lavender, patchouli, rosemary, sandalwood.

Greying hair

This is associated with hereditary factors and the ageing process. Poor nutrition and prolonged stress can also contribute. A well-balanced diet and stress-relieving measures, including Indian head massage, are useful preventative steps to take.

CARRIER OILS TO CHOOSE ⤜ olive, sesame.
ESSENTIAL OILS TO CHOOSE ⤜ Roman chamomile.

Hair loss

To a certain degree, hair loss is perfectly natural. We can shed as many as 100 hairs every day, under normal circumstances. Excessive hair loss, however, can often indicate a problem, such as hormonal imbalance, high stress levels, extreme dieting, or muscular tension that hinders the blood circulation to the scalp. Chemical treatments often exacerbate the problem. Indian head massage can help reduce hair loss by encouraging mental and physical relaxation and stimulating the circulation. Avoid using vigorous massage movements if the hair is very thin, and do not tug on the hair.

CARRIER OILS TO CHOOSE ⤜ mustard, sesame.
ESSENTIAL OILS TO CHOOSE ⤜ geranium, lavender, Roman chamomile, rosemary.

❧ If you are seriously concerned about the condition of your scalp or hair, consult your doctor who may suggest a referral to a trichologist – a specialist in treating hair problems.

☺ Nice or nasty?

Carrier and essential oils each have their own specific properties that should obviously be taken into account when choosing a lubricant for massage. However, the aroma is of particular importance. Give your massage partner the chance to "follow his nose" by offering a selection of appropriate oils – he will know instinctively which is best for him. If you or your partner strongly dislike a particular essential or carrier oil, do not use it. If you get the opportunity, you might like to try a few different oils before you buy. Pat a little on the inside of your wrist to get the best effect.

🖐 *The healing properties of essential oils have been known for many centuries. Hieroglyphics show that the ancient Egyptians used aromatic oils in their medicines. But the treatment system known as "aromatherapy" dates back only to the 1930s. This system was devised by the French cosmetic chemist Prof René Gattefosse who burnt his hand during an accident at his laboratory. He plunged his hand into the nearest bowl of liquid, which happened to be pure lavender oil, and the pain eased immediately. His hand healed quickly with minimal scarring and there was no sign of infection. He was so amazed by his discovery that he began a study of essential oils and called his findings "aromatherapie".*

☺ Carrier oils

There are many types of carrier oil. The most commonly used in Indian head massage are coconut, mustard, olive, sesame, sunflower, sweet almond and jojoba. The one to choose depends on special requirements, personal preference and whether the oil is tolerated by your massage partner's skin type.

Coconut *(Cocos nucifera)*

A cream-coloured semi-solid "oil" derived from the dried flesh of the coconut. It is very popular in the southern regions of India and is highly recommended for Indian head massage. It is a very light oil that can be used on its own, in combination with other carrier oils or blended with essential oils. It is virtually odourless and mixes well with fragranced oils. Coconut oil is highly refined, so many of its nutrients have been destroyed, but it has softening/moisturizing qualities.

A common ingredient in many hair and skin care preparations, coconut oil is suitable for all skin and hair types and gives hair a glossy shine. Solid coconut oil liquefies when warmed. Warm by placing the bottle near a radiator or in a jug of hot water for a few minutes. Pour as much as you need into a small bowl and stir before use. The oil left in the bottle will set as it cools and can be re-used in the same way. Fractionated or light coconut oil, which remains liquid at a wider range of temperatures, is also available.

CAUTIONS 🖐 **May irritate sensitive skin. Test before using by applying a little oil to the skin and waiting for any reaction. Do not use in cases of nut allergy.**

⬭ CASE STUDY ⬭

Sneezes and snuffles

Generally very fit and healthy, Tony, 74, started suffering from recurrent coughs and colds after the death of a good friend left him feeling rather low. It seemed that as soon as one infection cleared, he caught another. His skin looked dull and his hair lost its usual shine. "When the sniffles prevented me from going to my grandson's birthday party, I decided to do something about my health," he explained. "I went straight to our local health food store and was advised that stress may be lowering my immune system and that I should take some positive steps toward better health. One of the suggestions was a course of six Indian head massages.

"I liked the therapist as soon as I met her. She asked me lots of questions about my past and present health and lifestyle. I was pleased that she didn't put my health complaints down to old age but said that she would try to help my body rebalance itself. After the second session, I had another dreadful cold and didn't go for a couple of weeks, but as soon as I had recovered I went straight back to her. Within a couple of months I felt on great form. My skin looked better than ever and the oils gave my hair a lovely soft feel. I have a head massage about once a month now – it's a real treat and it certainly seems to keep the coughs and colds at bay. I have only had one cold in the last three months and that only lasted a few days."

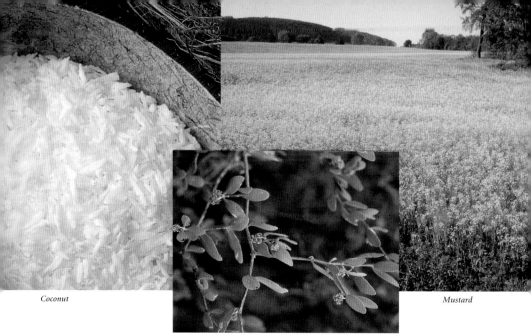

Coconut

Jojoba

Mustard

Jojoba *(Simmondsia chinensis)*

Jojoba (pronounced ho-ho-ba) oil comes from the fruit of an evergreen desert plant. It is extremely popular for skin and hair care and keeps well. It is an almost colourless, odourless liquid wax that is semi-solid at room temperature and solidifies when refrigerated. Excellent for all skin and hair types, jojoba oil contains vitamin E, protein and minerals, which are readily absorbed into the skin to give a moisturizing and nourishing effect.

It has a similar structure to sebum and combines with it to remove the dirt, grease and grime that can block pores. It can also help reduce muscular aches and pains. As it is very expensive, it is best to use jojoba in very small quantities – dilute it in the ratio 10:90 with another carrier oil.

CAUTIONS ℘ **Generally well tolerated.**

Mustard *(Brassica nigra)*

Mustard oil is a highly viscous, deep-yellow liquid, with a very pungent odour. It should not be confused with the non-greasy mustard essential oil, which is not suitable for home use. Mustard oil is popular in India, especially in West Bengal. The oil is extracted from the seeds of the plant, which has long been prized for its medicinal uses. The crushed seeds are used in Ayurvedic medicine to help aid digestion and stomach disorders. Mustard oil

is often used on its own as it has a powerful scent that does not mix well with essential oils. Mustard oil is very heavy and warming, a useful oil in the winter months. It helps stimulate the circulation of blood to the scalp and creates a warming, relaxing sensation that eases muscular tension, pain and stiffness. The best place to buy this oil is an Indian grocer's shop, where it is sold at a very reasonable price.

CAUTIONS ℘ **May cause some irritation on sensitive skins. Test before using by applying a little oil to the skin and waiting for any reaction.**

Olive *(Olea europea)*

Olive oil is a yellow-green, viscous liquid, derived from the fruits of the olive tree. It is readily available in most supermarkets and health food stores and is a useful oil for both massage and cooking. Look for products labelled "virgin" and "extra virgin", which contain high levels of unsaturated fatty acids and help moisturize dry skin and hair. Olive oil has similar properties to sesame oil and can help ease muscle pain and stiffness. It can be used on its own but, as it is rather thick and pungent, is best mixed 50:50 with another carrier oil, such as sweet almond.

CAUTIONS ℘ **Generally well tolerated.**

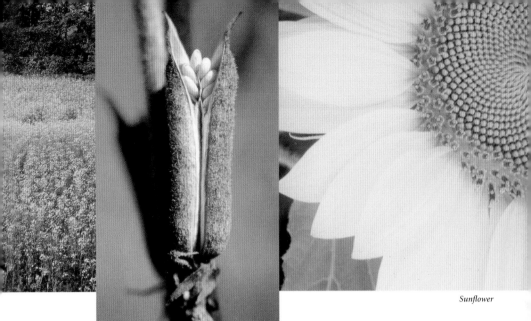

Sunflower

Sesame

Sesame *(Sesamum indicum)*

One of the most popular oils for massage in India, sesame oil is highly regarded in Ayurvedic medicine, both for internal and external use, and is reputed to prevent hair from turning grey. It is a golden-yellow, viscous liquid, derived from the untoasted seeds of the sesame plant, and has a light, slightly nutty aroma. Do not confuse it with the dark-brown sesame oil used in cooking. That oil is made from toasted sesame seeds and has a very strong smell.

Sesame oil is generally used on its own, but it can be mixed with other vegetable oils or blended with an essential oil such as sandalwood. Rich in vitamin E, iron and phosphorus, it is recommended for all skin and hair types and has a moisturizing, soothing, strengthening and balancing effect. Sesame oil can help ease muscular tension, pains and stiffness.

CAUTIONS ⚘ **May irritate sensitive skin (olive oil is an alternative). Test before using by applying a little oil on to the skin and waiting for any reaction.**

Sunflower *(Helianthus annus)*

This produces a light, pleasant oil that is useful to keep at home for both massage and culinary purposes. Look for unrefined, organically produced sunflower seed oil, which is available in many health food stores. It is a viscous, golden-yellow liquid, with a sweet, nutty aroma, which is derived from the seeds of the sunflower plant. Organic, unrefined sunflower oil is often used in body massage. It can be used on its own or blended with other oils. It mixes especially well with many essential oils, including frankincense and lavender. The unrefined, organic oil contains high amounts of unsaturated fatty acids and vitamins A, B, D and E and is suitable for all skin types, especially dry skin.

CAUTIONS ⚘ **Generally well tolerated.**

Sweet almond *(Prunus amygdalus)*

Sweet almond oil is extracted from the kernels of the sweet almond tree. It is a pale yellow, viscous liquid with a mild fragrance. The oil is very light and can be used on its own or as a blend. It is widely available, highly versatile and mixes well with most carrier oils and pure essential oils, especially Roman chamomile. Popular as a body massage oil, it is rich in unsaturated fatty acids and protein. It also contains vitamin A, some B vitamins and small amounts of vitamin E and D. Almond oil is often added to hair conditioners as it helps soften, moisturize and protect the hair. It is useful for easing muscular pain and stiffness and for aiding mobility.

CAUTIONS ⚘ **Well tolerated by most skin types. Do not use in cases of nut allergy. Do not confuse sweet almond oil with the oil made from bitter almonds, which has culinary applications but is never used in massage.**

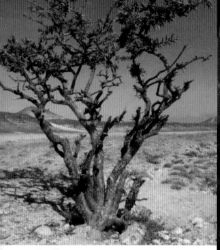

Frankincense

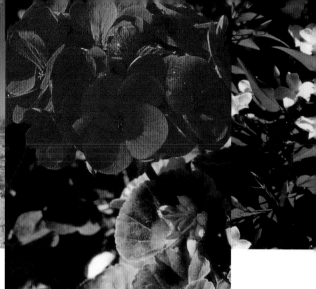

Geranium

◎ Recommended essential oils

These oils are safe to use at home so long as you dilute them with a carrier oil in the correct proportions and follow safety guidelines. To find out about other essential oils to use or avoid, and suitable dilutions, ask a qualified aromatherapist.

Frankincense *(Boswellia carteri)*

This is pale yellow or green with a warm, rich, sweet, spicy aroma. Frankincense was one of the three gifts presented to baby Jesus by the three Wise Kings. It was so highly regarded at the time that it was almost as precious as gold. It is a balancing, confidence-boosting oil that is often used in meditation as it aids concentration and focused thought. It is said to promote personal and spiritual growth and help break links with the past. Throughout history, frankincense has been burnt on altars and in temples during religious rituals and applied to the sick to disperse evil spirits.

Frankincense can aid relaxation and lift mental and physical lethargy. It helps induce deep, slow breathing, especially when used in an aromatherapy burner or sprinkled on a handkerchief, and so can help clear congestion of the sinuses and nasal passages. Suitable for all skin and hair types, it moisturizes dull, mature skin and acts as an astringent for oily skin and hair. Frankincense may also improve skin tone.

CAUTIONS ℘ **Generally well tolerated. Not to be used in pregnancy or for babies and children.**

Geranium *(Pelargonium graveolens)*

This is clear or pale-green with a fairly powerful sweet, refreshing, floral scent. It is a calming, strengthening and balancing oil that has a normalizing effect on the sebaceous glands, so making it useful for all skin conditions. Geranium is especially beneficial for improving the condition of very dry or very oily hair and skin. It is mildly astringent, a good skin cleanser and helpful for treating dandruff and head lice. Geranium oil is reputed to stimulate the blood circulation and boost the lymphatic system for speedy disposal of toxins and excess fluids from the body. It is often used to ease menstrual and menopausal tension and can help alleviate tension headaches.

Geranium is a versatile oil with a lovely scent. In Victorian England, geranium blooms were left at the sides of stairs so that the women's long skirts would brush against them and release the delightful perfume. The oil can be used to both soothe and uplift as it is a tonic for depression and has a calming influence on an over-active mind. Geraniums were traditionally grown in gardens and homes to keep evil spirits away. Try diffusing geranium oil into the atmosphere to create a harmonious mood in your home.

CAUTIONS ℘ **May irritate very sensitive skin. Test before using by applying a little diluted oil to the skin and waiting for any reaction. Not to be used in pregnancy or for babies and children.**

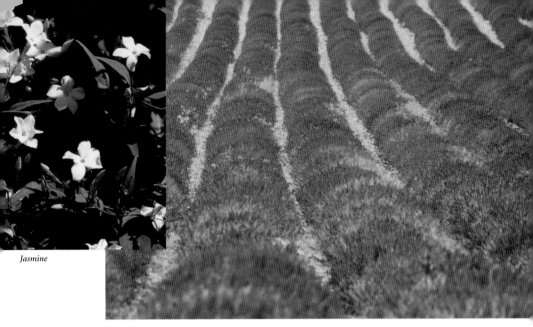

Jasmine

Lavender

Jasmine *(Jasminum officinalis)*

This is dark orange-brown with a rich, warm, heady, oriental aroma that tends to linger. Jasmine is known in India as "queen of the night" or "moonlight of the grove" because the scent of the delicate flowers is most intense at night. It is also called "king of perfumes" because of its exotic fragrance, which is popularly used in soaps, toiletries, cosmetics and perfumes. Jasmine is a very common ingredient in hair oils in India and is beneficial for all skin types, especially dry, sensitive skin. It also has an ancient reputation as an aphrodisiac – Cleopatra is said to have bathed in jasmine oil to help make her seem more desirable to her beloved Anthony.

Jasmine is a balancing oil that can be uplifting and relaxing, revitalizing and restorative. It helps create feelings of optimism, emotional warmth and self-confidence. It is often used to deepen and regulate breathing, and is useful in massage for relieving pain and relaxing tense muscles. Jasmine essential oil is very costly and so should be used sparingly. Alternatively use a pre-blended massage oil to experience the benefits of jasmine.

CAUTIONS ஜ **Use very sparingly – the aroma can be quite intoxicating – one drop in 30ml. It may cause irritation on very sensitive skins. Test before using by applying a little diluted oil to the skin and waiting for any reaction. Not to be used in pregnancy or for babies and children.**

Lavender *(Lavendula angustifolio)*

This is clear or faintly yellow with a light, fresh, floral aroma. Lavender is a balancing, normalizing oil with cleansing properties. The name derives from the Latin word *lavare* meaning "to wash". In Tudor times, women scattered lavender over their floors to cleanse and deodorize the rooms. Lavender oil can help regulate sebum production, so it is suitable for all skin and hair types. It is also useful for clearing dandruff, stimulating hair growth and repelling head lice.

On an emotional level, lavender helps induce feelings of composure, peace, contentment and tranquillity. It can be used to lift anxiety and depression, harmonize mood swings and ease tension headaches. A natural sedative, lavender oil is often used to prevent insomnia and aid restful sleep. Sprinkle two drops on a handkerchief and place inside your pillow at night. Lavender oil is also helpful in first aid for burns, stings, bites, bruises and wounds, as it has painkilling and antiseptic qualities that aid the healing process.

CAUTIONS ஜ **May not be tolerated well by people with hay fever, asthma or other allergic conditions. Not to be used in pregnancy or for babies and children.**

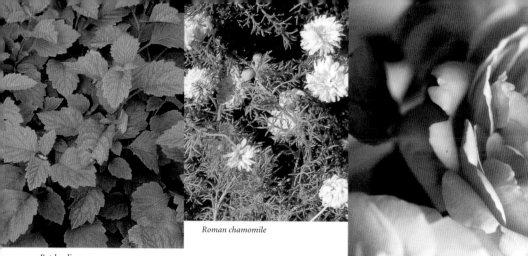

Roman chamomile

Patchouli

Rose

Patchouli *(Pogostemon cablin)*

This is dark-amber or reddish-brown with a rich, heavy, earthy, musky, sensuous aroma that people tend either to strongly like or dislike. Patchouli oil is often added to carrier oils for its exotic scent. It is highly evocative of the 1960s as it was the principal ingredient in many of the body perfumes of that era. In the East, dried patchouli leaves are used to perfume linen and fabrics, as the strong scent helps mask unpleasant odours and is thought to prevent the spread of disease and infection and to repel moths. Patchouli become popular in Britain during Victorian times, when cashmere shawls imported from India were a fashionable accessory. These shawls retained the lingering scent of the patchouli that was used for their transportation.

Patchouli is a good balancing oil that is used for many stress-related disorders. It can promote relaxation and help calm a troubled mind. It moisturizes dry, mature skin and aids the shedding of dead skin cells to create a fresher, younger appearance. Patchouli can help ease scalp problems such as dandruff and improve the condition of oily hair and skin. It is also reputed to be an aphrodisiac.

CAUTIONS ℘ The aroma is not to everyone's liking. Always use very sparingly. Not to be used in pregnancy or for babies and children.

Roman chamomile *(Chamaemelum nobile)*

Pale yellow in colour, Roman chamomile has a mild, sweet, slightly fruity aroma. The ancient Egyptians held chamomile in such high regard that the plant was declared sacred and dedicated to Ra, the sun god. It is a gentle, calming oil with a pleasant aroma that helps relax mind and body. A wonderful oil to use at the end of a long, tiring, stressful day, it can lift anxiety, doubts and worries. Roman chamomile is beneficial for any stress-related disorder including dull aches and pains, tension headaches and insomnia. It may help alleviate skin or hair problems associated with emotional stress. Commonly used in hair rinses, Roman chamomile has a lightening effect on fair hair and adds lustre and colour to grey hair. It is a good oil to choose for dry skin and hair conditions. It should be used very sparingly, however – one drop to 30ml (six teaspoons).

CAUTIONS ℘ It may cause irritation on sensitive skins. Test before using by applying a little diluted oil to the skin and waiting for any reaction. Not to be used in pregnancy or for babies and children.

Rose *(Rosa centifolia; Rosa damascena)*

So pale-yellow as to be almost colourless, rose has a deep, sweet floral smell. It is traditionally considered a "female" oil and associated with Venus, the Roman goddess of love and beauty. The Romans crowned their brides and bridegrooms with roses. Rose petals are collected at sunrise, when their scent is strongest, and processed within 24 hours. It takes around thirty roses to make a single drop of oil, which accounts for the high price. However, it is a very versatile and pleasant oil to use. It suits all skin and hair types and is a very effective moisturizer for dry, mature and sensitive skins. Rosewater is a mild, soothing, lightly perfumed tonic that can be used in massage if your partner has a very greasy scalp condition.

Rose aids meditation and relaxation and encour-

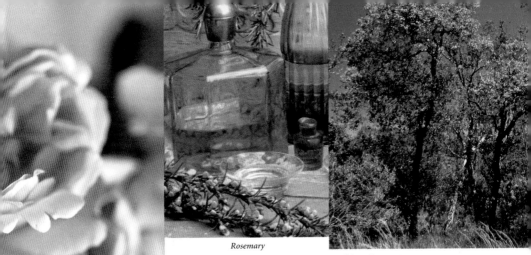

Rosemary

Sandalwood

ages mental alertness and optimism. It may help ease the symptoms of some menstrual disorders and is believed to stimulate the lymphatic system to remove excess fluid, toxins and waste products. Like jasmine, rose essential oil is expensive and should be used in small quatities. It is often sold ready diluted in a base oil, but do follow the instructions on the label very carefully to ensure that you use the correct amount. Alternatively use a pre-blended massage oil.

CAUTIONS 🌿 **Generally well tolerated but may cause a reaction in some very sensitive people. Use one drop per 30ml of carrier oil. Test before using by applying a little diluted oil to the skin. Not to be used in pregnancy or for babies and children.**

Rosemary *(Rosmarinus officinalis)*

This is clear or very pale yellow with a strong, fresh, herbal aroma. Rosemary has long been associated with improving brain power and mental alertness. The Greeks used to put twigs of rosemary in their hair to help boost concentration during examinations, while Ophelia in Shakespeare's Hamlet refers to its memory-enhancing powers: "There's rosemary, that's for remembrance." It is an excellent oil to diffuse in an aromatherapy burner while studying or meditating as it lifts mental fatigue and clears the head.

Rosemary is an invigorating, energizing oil that can help stimulate the blood circulation to the scalp and so improve the condition of the hair and promote its growth. It is said to enhance the colour of dark hair. It has an astringent action that helps tighten skin and harmonize greasy hair and skin. Rosemary is a useful oil to treat dandruff and protect against head lice.

CAUTIONS 🌿 **May irritate sensitive skin. Test before using by applying a little diluted oil to the skin and waiting for any reaction. Do not use if the person suffers from epilepsy or high blood pressure. Not to be used in pregnancy or for babies and children.**

Sandalwood *(Santalum album)*

This is clear or pale-green with a sweet, woody, sensual, distinctly oriental aroma that lingers for a long time. Sandalwood is included in the ancient Ayurvedic texts as an important therapeutic plant. In its powdered form, sandalwood is a popular incense and has been used as an aid to meditation for at least four thousand years. The wood was traditionally used in India for sacred carvings and in the building of ancient temples. Sandalwood trees are protected in India and regarded as the property of the Indian Government. One of the oldest known scented materials, the aroma of sandalwood eases nervous tension and anxiety and creates a feeling of emotional calm and well-being, making it a useful aid to relaxation and self-healing. Sandalwood is also reputed to be an aphrodisiac and is said to boost the immune system and induce restful sleep.

The diluted essential oil can help soothe and soften dry, mature skin and acts as a mild astringent for oily skin and hair. It is known to help relieve itching and so may ease the irritation caused by dandruff.

CAUTIONS 🌿 **May not be well-tolerated by people with very sensitive skins. Look for the highest quality oil, which comes from the Mysore region of India. Test before using by applying a little diluted oil to the skin and waiting for any reaction. Not to be used in pregnancy or for babies and children.**

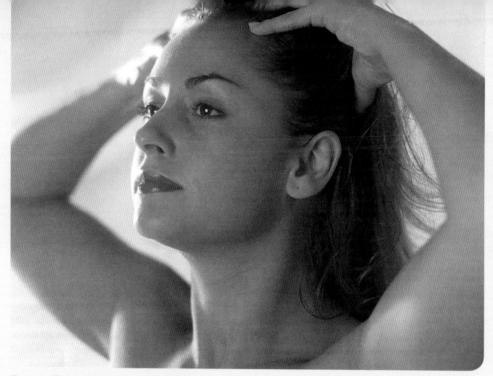

Treat yourself to a head massage.

☺ Self-massage

Follow the tradition of Indian women and give yourself an oily scalp massage once a week to encourage your locks to grow strong, shiny and more manageable. Massage stimulates the flow of blood and lymph through the scalp, bringing fresh supplies of oxygen and nutrients to the hair follicles and removing any toxins and waste products that could hinder healthy growth. Natural vegetable oils can help cleanse, nourish and improve the condition of your scalp and moisturize, strengthen and protect your hair, helping to promote a glossy sheen.

There is no need to shampoo your hair first unless it is very dirty. If you wash your hair before massage, towel it dry before you begin. Comb through with a wide-tooth comb.

✿ Scalp massage with oil is very beneficial for dry hair or hair that has been treated with chemicals. However, do wait a week after a perm or other treatment using chemicals to allow your hair to settle. If you have any doubts, ask your hairdresser.

Choose an oil or blend of oils to suit your hair type and mood. Rub some oil into your hands and then, working from the front of your head to the back, stroke it evenly all over your scalp. Now place your hands in a claw-like position on your head, fingers well spread-out, and make small rotations with the pads of your fingers and thumbs all over your scalp. The pressure should be firm but comfortable. Feel your scalp moving beneath your fingers. Keep your fingers moving so you do not spend too long working on the same area.

Self-massage can make your arms ache, so try resting your elbows on a table. Continue for at least five minutes until you have covered the whole of your head. Include the hair line and temples where muscles tend to get very tense, so restricting the flow of blood to the hair follicles. You may also like to try some of the other movements from the step-by-step suggestions in the following chapters. Finish with some gentle stroking movements to soothe and relax. Cover your head with a warm towel and rest. It is best to keep the oil on your head for at least half an hour before washing to gain maximum benefits.

Top-to-toe massage

A weekly full-body massage using organic vegetable oils is an integral part of Ayurvedic recommendations for a long and healthful life. It is obviously not as enjoyable as being massaged by someone else, but it is a very good way of keeping your skin and hair in good condition and also of giving you time to get in touch with your body. This routine is quick, simple and effective. Use an unrefined carrier oil or a special massage blend. Sesame oil is generally favoured for a full body massage in Ayurvedic medicine, but you may prefer to choose an oil with a more fragrant aroma.

- Undress and sit or stand on a towel you have spread out on the floor in a warm and comfortable place. Apply your chosen oil all over the body. Start with your head and massage your scalp with small, circular strokes.

- Now move downward, covering your entire body: face and arms first, then chest, legs and feet. Use the flat of your hand, not just your fingertips, to perform upward massage strokes, directing the venous blood flow back to the heart. Apply more vigorous strokes on your head, arms and legs and moderate pressure to the rest of your body. Be gentle over your face and abdomen. Use long strokes on the straight areas of your body, such as arms and legs, and large circular strokes over rounded areas and joints, such as your elbows and hips.

- At the end of the massage, sit quietly for a few minutes and practise a relaxation technique (see page 60). If possible, leave the oil on your skin for at least twenty minutes before showering.

- If you do not have time for a full-body massage, just apply a lightly fragranced carrier oil to your face, neck and feet. This will only take a couple of minutes. Undress and wrap a warm towel around you. Sit on another towel laid out on the floor. Apply the oil to your forehead, temples, ears and neck in gentle soothing strokes. Now massage oil into the soles of your feet. Sit quietly for a few minutes before washing your feet in warm water. This is a very relaxing massage to have in the evening, just before bedtime.

Shirodhara

An Ayurvedic treatment session often ends with a luxuriously relaxing technique known as Shirodhara, pictured below. After a head massage, warm sesame oil is dripped over the centre of the forehead in a slow, steady stream. In Ayurveda, the middle of the forehead marks the position of the "third eye", an area of great spiritual significance. Shirodhara can continue for up to an hour and helps lift depression and mental fatigue.

Ayurvedic treatment in Sri Lanka.

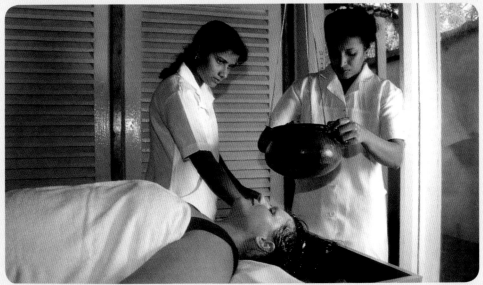

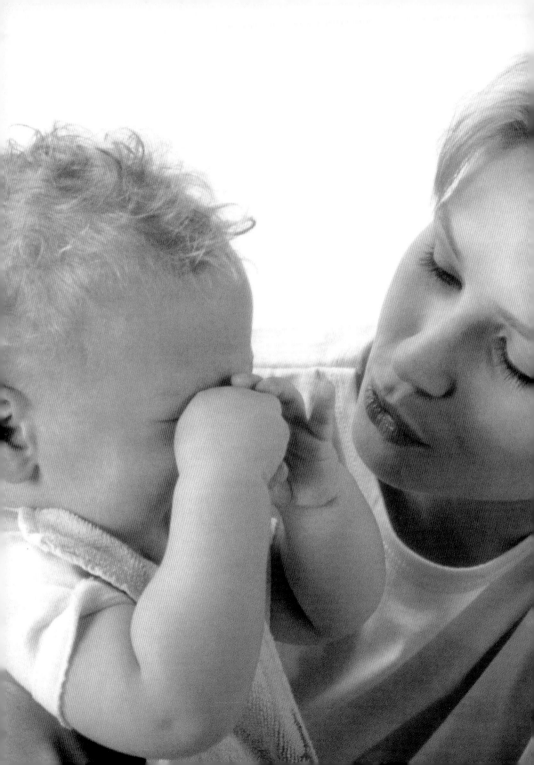

CHAPTER FOUR

INDIAN HEAD MASSAGE TECHNIQUES

MASSAGE IS A BASIC, nurturing instinct that we all share. We use our natural healing power of touch in our everyday lives, often without realizing it. Think how we instinctively rub a sore spot to ease the pain or offer comforting strokes to reassure an anxious child. These are all basic forms of massage that have been practised all over the world since ancient times. Indian head massage develops these intuitive skills into a flowing sequence of therapeutic movements.

In India, the skills of massage are passed down through the generations. Children, who are massaged regularly from a very young age, instinctively pick up the techniques through their own experience. When they grow up and have children of their own they, in turn, share them with their offspring. Each person naturally acquires their own particular style. This can be readily adapted to suit the individual by including favourite movements or varying the speed and pressure of strokes in order to relax or stimulate.

✌ Types of massage stroke

Massage of any kind can be classed as the manipulation of the body's soft tissues – the skin, fat and muscle and the connective tissue that holds the organs and underlying structures in place. It involves a series of movements using the hands. Each movement is applied in a particular way in order to have a specific effect on the area being massaged. Once you appreciate the essential differences between the actions and the benefits of the various manipulations, you can try other combinations of strokes and devise your own safe and effective routines to suit different occasions.

> *With practice, you will learn to use your hands to detect factors that will influence your style of massage, such as the tightness of muscles, areas of tension, amount of fat and skin texture.*

For ease of understanding, the different rubbing, squeezing, pressing, kneading, patting and tapping movements are classified by means of the widely recognized terminology of Swedish-style massage. This system was developed by physiologist Per Henrik Ling in the early 1800s and is now taught internationally to massage students. The main movements are stroking, effleurage, petrissage, frictions and tapotement. It is not easy to learn these movements from a book. Do remember, however, that the secret of a good massage is in applying each stroke with care and affection to make your partner feel nurtured and secure.

> *Do not worry if you feel clumsy or awkward when you start to practise these different techniques. You will be pleasantly surprised at how quickly your movements begin to flow.*

Stroking

Stroking is particularly effective on the face and scalp. These areas are well supplied with a mass of sensory nerve endings that quickly respond to touch and can strongly influence the way you feel, both mentally and physically. Soft stroking has an almost soporific effect on your mind and body, while faster, more energetic stroking will revitalize you, lifting lethargy and weariness. An Indian head massage often combines both gentle and brisk stroking to relax and refresh. A massage usually begins with gentle stroking in any direction to apply the oil to the scalp and help your partner get used to the sensation of touch. Gentle stroking is a slow, light and superficial gliding

movement designed to soothe and relax the sensory nerves. It is the kind of smooth, rhythmical, repetitive action we naturally use to pacify a baby or stroke a pet. Your hands are open and supple so they mould to the shape of the part being massaged.

Brisk stroking or rubbing is widely used in Indian head massage. However, in the West, we tend to prefer a lighter touch rather than the more powerful approach adopted by Indian masseurs using traditional methods. Your hands work very briskly over the surface of the skin using short, invigorating movements back and forth in any direction – rather like rubbing out a mistake with an eraser. Wrists are flexible, with fingers held quite straight. Depending on the size of the area being massaged, you can use the palm, side or heel of the hand, or the pads of several fingers. Rubbing stimulates the blood supply to the local blood vessels and warms the area. This is, in fact, our natural response when we feel chilly – we rub the cold area briskly to generate warmth.

> *You can give a very pleasurable massage by using stroking and effleurage movements alone. Change the effect by altering the pressure, speed, direction and length of stroke. Try it on yourself to feel how different variations have their own special impact.*

Stroking can be soft and gentle to promote a calming and soothing effect or brisk and energetic to revitalize.

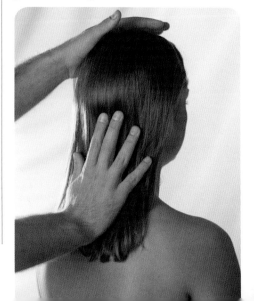

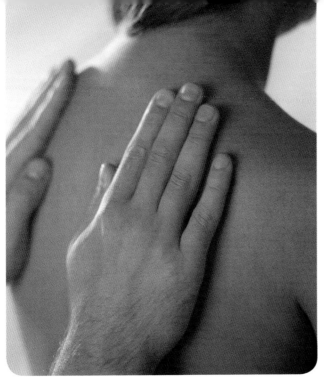

Effleurage is the use of pressure to create a light or firm stroke.

Effleurage

This is a similar movement to stroking but is generally a firmer, smoothing action. It is like the relaxed hands of a sculptor moulding the contours of a piece of clay to shape a statue. Effleurage helps improve the superficial blood circulation – the stroke follows the direction of the venous flow back to the heart. If the stroke is directed toward the nearest set of lymph nodes, it also aids lymphatic drainage, so helping the body rid itself of toxins. Keep your wrists flexible and your hands supple and flowing. Your pressure should increase slightly toward the end of the stroke and then return with a light touch, maintaining some hand or finger contact at all times. On larger areas, such as the upper back, use the palm of one or both hands. On smaller areas, use the soft pads of your thumbs or fingertips.

Slow effleurage, using moderate or light pressure, flows on naturally from gentle stroking and helps prepare the soft tissues for subsequent deeper massage movements. The underlying muscles are warmed and relaxed, thereby gradually easing any pain or soreness and allowing more freedom of movement. Once the muscles start to lose their tension, a faster effleurage action with deeper pressure can be uplifting and energizing.

✦ Practise whenever you get the opportunity. Hopefully, you should have no shortage of volunteers. The more you practise the movements, the more natural they become. Try massaging people of different builds, hair types and ages in order to broaden your range of experience.

Petrissage

This is a deeper movement than effleurage and so is mainly used on the muscles and fleshier areas. It is also called kneading because, as the name implies, the action is rather like kneading dough. The soft tissues are picked up and separated from the underlying structure and then compressed and released. Throughout this movement, your fingers or whole hands act like a pump, working on the deeper blood and lymph vessels to force blood and lymph back to the heart and squeeze out any toxins that have accumulated in the tissue spaces. The movement is slow and rhythmic with a deep but appropriate pressure. Be careful not to pinch and avoid working too long in one area, as this can cause discomfort and even bruising on sensitive skin.

You may find it helpful to refer back to this chapter when you are reading the step-by-step instructions for different strokes and routines.

As with stroking and effleurage, your shoulders and wrists should be relaxed and your hands supple and moulded to the shape of the area being massaged. Your hands do not glide over the surface of the skin but press much deeper to move the skin against the soft tissues below. You will be able to feel the underlying tissues moving and feel any nodules of tension or tight adhesions as you roll the fleshy mass with your hands. Kneading is a circular movement with an increase in pressure on the upward half of the circle and a decrease on the downward half. Once the movement is complete, your hand moves smoothly to the next part so that the rhythm of the massage is not disturbed.

You can vary the kneading movements by using the palm and fingers of one or both hands, or the fleshy pads of fingers or thumbs. In an Indian head massage, most kneading movements are performed with the fingers or thumbs.

Petrissage is a deeper, kneading movement made on the muscles.

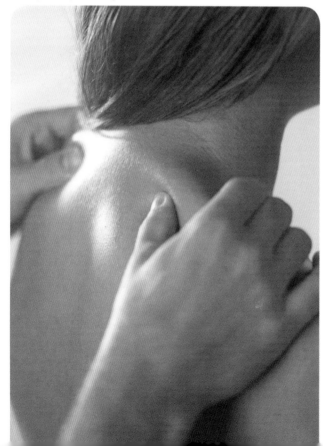

CHECKLIST

Benefits of petrissage

- The rhythmical compression and relaxation of the hands mimics a pump to boost the flow of deoxygenated blood back to the heart. This speeds up the removal of waste products and encourages the flow of arterial blood carrying oxygen and nutrients to the muscles and underlying structures.

- The pumping action also improves the flow of lymph to the nearest set of lymph nodes, so waste products and excess tissue fluid are quickly flushed out.

- Deep kneading is very effective in aiding blood and lymph circulation in muscle fibres, so reducing pain, tension and stiffness. The improved blood supply and lymphatic drainage provide the conditions necessary for faster recovery. The area is also warmed, which helps soothe and relax tense muscles.

- Compression movements help break down and loosen any adhesions or tension nodules in the muscle fibres.

- All kneading movements stimulate the sebaceous glands to secrete.

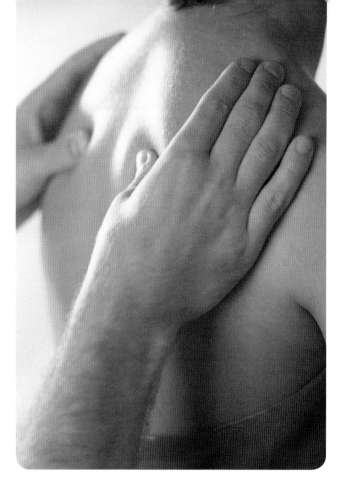

Frictions are deep, penetrating movements made with the pads of the fingers or thumbs.

Frictions

Frictions are small, deep, penetrating movements generally carried out using the pads of the fingers or thumbs. The skin moves over the underlying structures so that one layer of tissue is pressed firmly against another. The frictions used in Indian head massage are circular, progressively increasing the pressure as you move deeper and deeper, or static, pressing on a single point. Circular frictions are an entirely different movement from finger and thumb kneading, where a mass of muscle tissue is massaged, with the pressure increasing on the upward half of the circle and decreasing on the downward half. Frictions are smaller, more specific movements localized on a particular spot with a gradual increase in pressure.

Keep your fingers firm, pressing deeply by using your body weight. You can add more weight by placing one hand on top of the other or using two fingers or thumbs. Once you have completed the movement, usually after three seconds of static friction or after three complete circular movements, lift your fingers or thumbs and glide on to an adjacent area. Frictions are especially beneficial in targeting trouble-spots. There is often a sense of great relief as muscular tension dissipates.

Tense muscles can be very tender, so frictions should only be applied once the area has been warmed with more superficial movements. Start gently and increase the pressure. It may help to ask your partner to exhale as you apply the pressure and inhale as you relax the pressure. Do not work the same area for any length of time and stop at once if your partner experiences discomfort. Finish by soothing the area with stroking or effleurage.

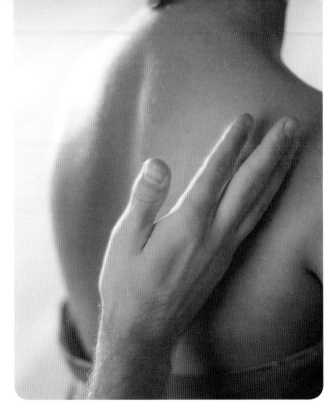

The rhythmical tapotement movements need to be practiced.

Tapotement

These movements are also known as percussion. They involve striking or tapping the skin and then releasing in the same rapid, rhythmical way as using a percussion instrument. Keep your wrists flexible and use your hands or fingers alternately to tap the skin with a light, springy movement. Your hands or fingers bounce back as soon as they land on the skin. It is best to start and finish each sequence of tapotement with a lighter pressure to avoid an abrupt shock. When using these more vigorous movements, start and finish with stroking and effleurage to warm and prepare the area and then afterward to soothe the sensory nerve endings and aid the flow of any excess blood or lymph back to the heart.

Tapotement movements for Indian head massage include tapping and hacking. Tapping is performed with the tips of fingers bouncing rhythmically up and down – rather like raindrops falling lightly on the ground. Hacking is performed with the sides of the hands in a series of short, sharp taps. Begin hacking with your hands pushed together. Now take your elbows away from your sides and separate your hands. Keep

your wrists flexible and move your forearms down and up so that the outer borders of your hands strike the area alternately. It is not a chopping action using both hands at the same time. Your hands move one after the other – strike, release, strike, release quickly and briefly in a brisk rhythmical way. The movement comes from the elbows while your upper arms remain still. You should always work around any obviously bony areas and avoid using tapotement on a very thin person. Never hack on a very sensitive area such as the spine or face.

It takes practice to get the rhythm of hacking. If the rhythm is unbalanced it can be a very irritating movement to receive. Before you start on a person, practise hacking whenever you can on different surfaces – a cushion, a kitchen work surface or a desk. Start slowly and increase speed without losing the rhythm.

Practise these movements individually before you put them all together. Get constructive criticism from a willing partner or work on yourself to get a feel for the effect of the different manipulations.

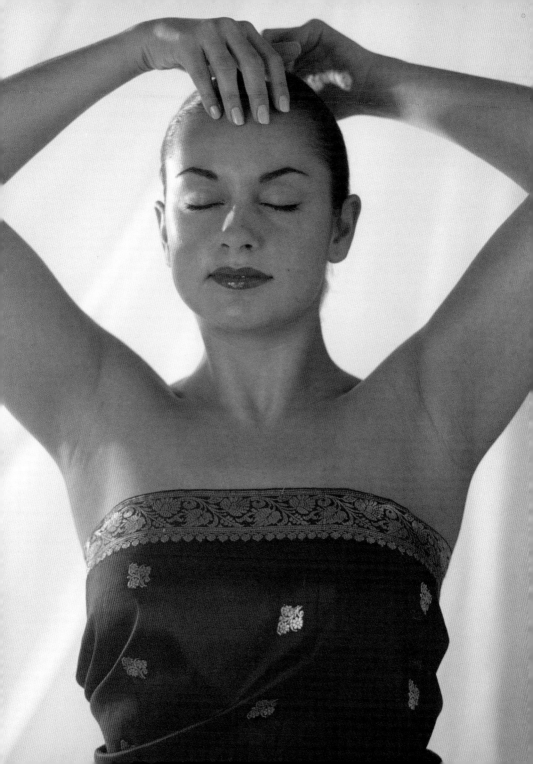

✆ Massage guidelines

The following guidelines will help ensure a safe and effective massage.

✦ Always check that your partner is not suffering any conditions that may make massage inadvisable (see page 65).

✦ **Massage should not cause severe sharp pain or discomfort. Stop if your partner feels dizzy, sick or nauseous. Ask your partner to tell you if she finds any strokes painful or in any way distressing so you can stop and quickly move on. Be guided by your partner. Never massage directly over the spine or any bony protrusions. Do not hack on the face.**

✦ Make every effort to ensure your partner feels nurtured, cosseted and secure. Warm towels are a lovely extra. Spend time checking your partner's comfort and asking about any massage strokes that she particularly enjoys. Start with gentle, slow, caring strokes to relax and spread the oil. Slowly increase the pressure and speed.

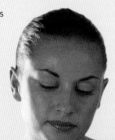

Make sure your partner is comfortable and relaxed.

✦ Be aware of your partner's body language. Around 70 per cent of all communication is by means of non-verbal messages and gestures. Take note of any flinching or stiffening that might indicate discomfort or unease. Similarly, look out for signs of evident enjoyment, such as relaxed breathing and a gentle purr of pleasure. Adapt your massage accordingly.

✦ Try not to chat too much. This will not only hinder your concentration but also upset the flow of the massage. Limit talking to a brief discussion of comfort, warmth and pressure. Background music can help discourage talk. At the start of the massage, advise your partner to let her mind empty. Discourage her from smoking, reading or looking around. Instead, you should encourage her to give herself totally to the massage. If her mind is still over-active, suggest that she focuses on the music, a favourite colour or the rhythm of your breathing.

✦ **Do not massage for too long or too often. A massage of the scalp can be very powerful and stimulating – a weekly session lasting around half an hour is generally considered ideal. Be wary of being too rough, or working on the same area for too long, as this may lead to bruising of the skin or weakening of the hair roots.**

✦ Choose a time when you are both in the mood for massage and there is little likelihood of being interrupted. Never try to coerce an unwilling partner, or rush a massage. If necessary, postpone the session until you will both be more receptive to the benefits.

✦ **Be aware of your posture. You do not want to end up with aches and pains! Stand with your feet apart to maintain a good balance. You can then use your weight to increase the pressure. Keep your back straight and your shoulders relaxed.**

- If you feel yourself slumping, make a conscious effort to lengthen your spine and neck. When you need to reduce your height, always bend your knees rather than your back, or kneel, if you find it more comfortable. Do not remain in one place, but move around the chair so you do not need to strain to reach. Take deep, long and regular breaths to help calm and relax you both.

- Maintain continuity. An Indian head massage should be as fluid and rhythmical as possible, flowing smoothly between soothing, gentle movements and brisk, more vigorous movements. Try not to stop and start. If you forget a movement, improvise. Your massage partner will not notice. If you need more oil, keep one hand, or at least an elbow, in contact with your partner's skin for as long as you can. Never jerk both hands away at once as this can be surprisingly disconcerting.

- Judge the depth of the pressure. Most people prefer a fairly firm massage around their shoulders and scalp and a lighter pressure on the face, but everyone has different physical needs and a different pain threshold. Always check with your partner – if the pressure is too deep it can be painful. If your touch is too light it can be rather irritating. Either way, if the pressure is wrong the muscles will tense up in response. If an area is ticklish, try increasing the depth of the pressure or simply move on. Younger, fitter people tend to like firmer pressure, while older people and children tend to prefer a lighter massage. Decrease your pressure over sensitive or bony areas, to avoid causing pain. Be gentle over the face so you do not drag the skin. Increase your pressure over larger muscles and fatty areas which may need some extra work.

- Massage can be applied to relax and soothe, or to stimulate and invigorate. As a general rule, softer, slower strokes are calming, while faster, brisker movements are energizing.

- If you are using oils, always let your partner express a preference.

- Give your partner the chance to sit quietly at the end of the massage. This allows time to make a gentle transition back to the real world.

Use fluid and rhythmical movements for a successful massage.

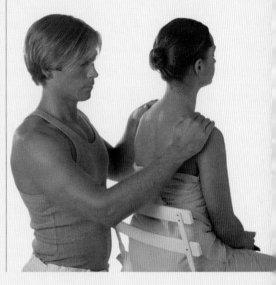

CASE STUDY

Harmony at home

Jessica, 15, says Indian head massage has helped improve her relationship with her mother. "When Mum first started at college she kept asking to practise on me," she explained. "At first I wouldn't let her near my hair but I eventually gave in – so long as she didn't use any of her oils. I'm really glad that I did. It's hard to put into words the effect that it has – but it is amazing. I don't understand quite why or how you can feel so different in such a short time, but you do.

"I didn't really notice any change until after the third or fourth massage. It was quite nice to be massaged but that was it. Then I think I started relaxing a bit more, letting myself enjoy the massage. And I realized how much better I felt in myself afterward. Sort of happier and more confident. Mum has been giving me Indian head massages on and off for about six months now and we both notice that I don't get nearly so uptight as I used to – little things don't get me down so much. I feel much closer to Mum. I let her use oil now, and I'm sure my hair is less tangly and more bouncy."

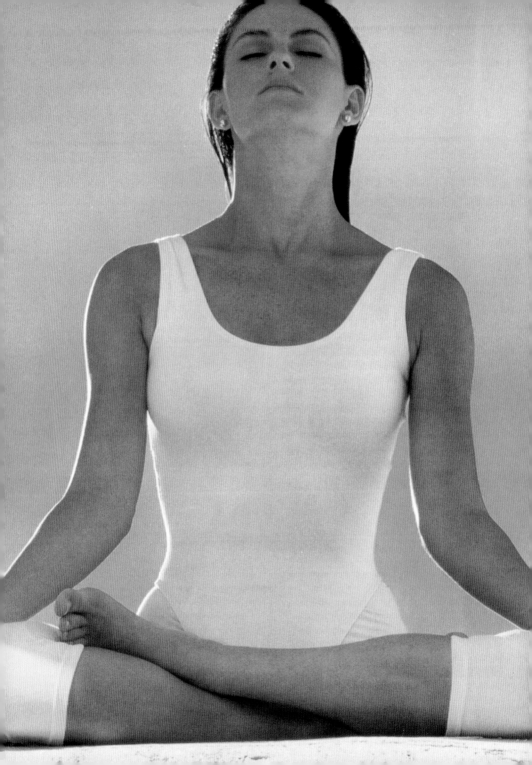

CHAPTER FIVE

THE ART OF RELAXATION

THOROUGH PREPARATION before an Indian head massage is very valuable. This includes making sure that both you and your massage partner are in a calm, relaxed state of mind, the atmosphere of the room is conducive to massage and everything you need is close at hand. It is also important to ensure that your partner is not suffering from a condition that might make massage inadvisable.

☙ Relaxation techniques

Practising simple relaxation exercises before an Indian head massage can help your massage partner to enjoy a smooth transition from the hurly-burly of everyday life into a state of deep physical and mental ease. The chances are, however, that just telling him to "relax" will only induce hunched shoulders and furrowed brows, so it may be helpful to offer some practical suggestions. The following relaxation techniques also offer useful strategies for managing stressful situations with inner peace, composure and serenity. Practise these exercises on your own and then with your massage partner.

A breath of fresh air

Breathing is a good reflection of your state of mind. When feeling stressed, your breathing tends to become shallow, uneven, rapid and noisy. This upsets the balance of carbon dioxide and oxygen within your body, which, in turn, leads to further physical and psychological tension. When relaxed, your breathing is deep, even, slow and quiet. The beautifully relaxed breathing of a child who is fast asleep in bed has an instantly calming effect. A good way of slowing your breathing is to focus on each breath as it enters and leaves your body – flowing smoothly and continuously in a balanced way.

1   Sit in a comfortable position, or lie on the floor, with your hands by your sides. Breathe in deeply through your nose, drawing the breath right down to your abdomen. Your abdomen should expand first, followed by your chest.

2   Rest for a moment, while still holding the breath, and then allow the breath to flow out, slowly and gently. At first, it may help you to rest your right hand on your abdomen until you get used to the feel of the movement.

3   Repeat this several times, concentrating on trying to empty the lungs. Practise this breathing technique for five minutes. If you sense that your breathing is becoming erratic, slow it down. Notice how much better you feel afterward.

Step-by-step relaxation

Once you start to feel the difference between tense and relaxed muscles, you will instantly recognize when you are holding tension and can then make a conscious effort to relax and let go. You can try the following full sequence, or a shortened version, wherever you are – watching television, having a bath, while waiting for a train, or just before

an important meeting. You will find that it eases aches and pains and gives you a greater sense of control and self-confidence. This progressive relaxation exercise involves deliberately tensing and relaxing the different muscles in your body.

1   Sit or lie comfortably. Loosen any tight clothing. Breathe deeply and evenly, allowing the breath to flow to all parts of your body.

2   Tense the muscles in your forehead, hold for a count of five and then relax, releasing any tension and enjoying the feeling of letting go.

3   Now concentrate on tensing the muscles of your eyes, cheeks and mouth (a most unflattering expression!), hold for a count of five and then release.

4   Continue with your neck and shoulders, arms and fingers, first tensing and then releasing the muscles. Hunch your shoulders and then let them drop and relax – feel the tension easing. Grip your fingers tightly and then let go. It is a wonderful feeling.

5   Continue this movement working down your body, tensing, holding and relaxing the muscles.

Visualizing paradise

Visualizations are really just formalized daydreams. They can help you to switch off from the daily grind and enter a more serene mental state.

1   Sit comfortably and quietly. Breathe in and out deeply and evenly. Close your eyes and imagine that you are in a pleasant location full of happy memories and joyful associations. You might be on a beach, or in the depth of the country among the miracles of nature. Spend a few quiet minutes in this place.

2   Use all your senses to recreate the feeling of being there, both physically and emotionally. What can you see? What sounds can you hear? What can you smell or taste? Are you lying, sitting or standing? What can you feel against your skin? When thoughts start to wander, return to this special scene.

3   Slowly open your eyes and gradually re-enter the real world.

Simple meditation

The following meditation is a useful aid to relaxation. Begin by meditating for a couple of minutes every day and gradually build up to twenty minutes once or twice a day. Before you start, make sure that you will not be disturbed. Set an alarm clock if you are concerned about the time.

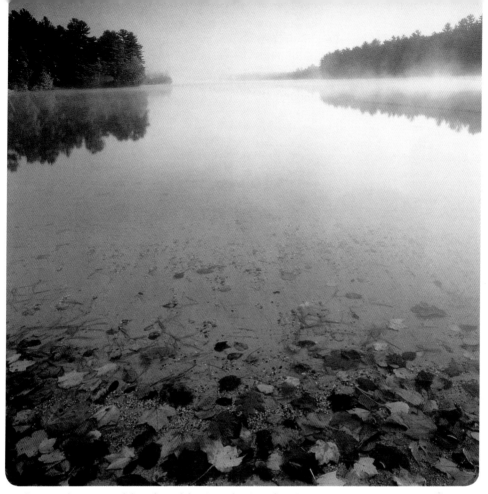

Visualize a scene that conjures up feelings of warmth, happiness, relaxation and serenity.

1 Sit in a comfortable position. close your eyes and breathe in through your nose. Allow the breath to reach deep down into your lungs. Exhale slowly through your mouth. Remain still and quiet for a few moments, listening to the regular flow of your breath.

2 Feel your body relaxing completely. Start with the muscles of your scalp and face and slowly work down your body, releasing all the tension as you go.

3 Focus on a single word, such as "one" or "peace". Keep repeating it aloud or to yourself. If you prefer, you can focus your attention on a favourite colour. Think of the colour in its lightest form. Picture it getting darker and richer, swirling around and forming exquisite patterns. Gradually, let the colour drain away so that it becomes paler and paler until it disappears altogether.

At first, all sorts of thoughts may keep coming into your head. Acknowledge them, but then go back to concentrating on your chosen word or colour.

It takes practice to empty the mind of stimulating thoughts or niggling problems – but it is well worth the effort. A few minutes of inner silence on a regular basis is a truly exquisite experience that has lasting benefits for physical and emotional health and well-being. Try to set aside a certain time each day to relax the tensions in your body and allow your mind to be free from daily pre-occupations. You will soon start to feel noticeably happier, calmer and more fulfilled. If you find it does not work at first, do not force yourself or try too hard. Wait a couple of days and then try again.

Feeling centred

Stress can affect your massage. Think how someone in a bad mood can alter the whole atmosphere at home or work. If you are tense and irritable, you can easily pass it on to others. If you are upset, worried or ill, your massage partner may well pick up on your negative mood. There is also a risk that you could take out your frustrations with excessively vigorous movements. And it works the other way, too. When you are feeling low or vulnerable, you are also more receptive to your massage partner's moods. To help make an Indian head massage a positive experience for the both of you, aim to get into a tranquil and confident frame of mind. This is often referred to as being "centred" or "grounded". Try to create your own personal space so you can distance your emotions from those of your massage partner. The following sequence can help.

1 Take five deep breaths. As you breathe in, feel that you are absorbing calm and peace. Breathe out slowly, letting all your anxieties and tensions flow from you. Some people like to picture themselves surrounded by a strong bubble that protects them from any unpleasant or stressful thoughts or feelings.

2 Another way of detaching yourself and developing a deep sense of calm is to stand quietly for a few minutes with your feet firmly on the floor. Imagine that you are a tree with golden roots growing deep down into the ground. Picture these golden roots giving you strength and stability.

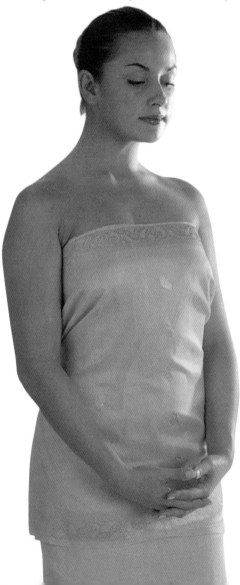

Helping hands

When giving a massage, you communicate with your massage partner mainly through your hands. They need to be warm, soft and supple to ensure a caring touch, yet well co-ordinated and flexible enough to perform the variety of massage movements so effectively used in Indian head massage. Aim to keep your nails clean, trimmed and filed to avoid scratching the skin. If possible, it is best not to wear nail polish when massaging as this could chip off, causing discomfort, and may even trigger an allergic reaction. Odours can linger on the hands, so make sure they do not smell of nicotine or the meal you have been preparing. Wear rubber gloves when chopping onions or garlic.

When you are trying to relax and reassure your partner, the warmth of your hands matters more than you may realize. The touch of cold hands can give a nasty shock and may cause muscles to tense – think what it feels like to jump into an icy shower. So, before you begin, especially if your hands tend to get very cold, rub them briskly together, or immerse them in warm water for a few minutes.

With practice, you will find that your hands become stronger and more flexible. Meanwhile, the following hand and finger exercises can help reduce muscle fatigue in your hands and improve your technique. Repeat them several times a day, whenever you get a free moment, and perform them as a warm-up routine just before giving a massage.

1 Remove all jewellery from your hands and wrists. Hold your hands at chest level and shake them from your wrist for a count of ten. Keep the movement loose and vigorous.

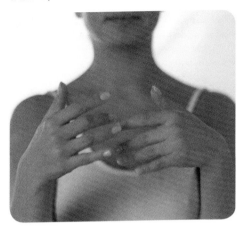

2 Make fists with both hands and rotate them from the wrist in a circular movement ten times. Repeat in the reverse direction.

3 Separate your fingers and thumbs and stretch them out as far they will reach. Hold for a count of ten. Repeat three times.

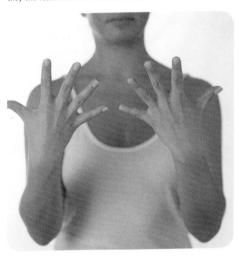

4 Put your hands on a flat surface with the palms facing downward. First, lift your thumbs, then each finger in turn, as though playing a piano. Return to the starting position by placing your little fingers on the surface, followed by each individual finger. Repeat three times.

5 Place the palms of your hands together and press one hand firmly against the other. Hold for a couple of seconds and then release. Repeat ten times.

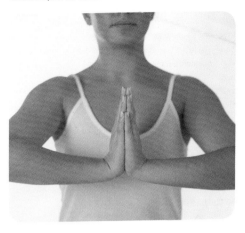

6 Hold a small rubber ball in your hand. Squeeze it as hard as you can, for a count of ten, and then release. Do this three times, then repeat, this time holding the ball in the other hand. This is also a great stress-busting exercise.

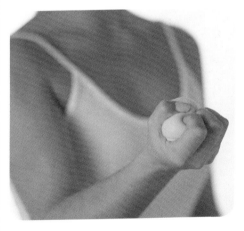

✿ The use of massage oils should keep your hands well mois-turized. You may find that they are now in better condition than they have ever been before.

✺ Creating a healing atmosphere

The art of relaxation is in creating a warm, comfortable and peaceful environment. It is worthwhile spending time and thought on getting the room fully prepared well in advance so you can both relax and enjoy the whole experience in tranquil surroundings.

Preparation

Get ready beforehand. For example, make sure you have plenty of towels and sufficient oil. Lay everything out ready so that, once you have started, you will not need to leave the room or search in drawers. Check the room temperature. The room should be warm enough to encourage deep physical and mental relaxation without being too stifling. Even if you get pretty hot and sticky while massaging, your massage partner's body temperature can start to drop as tension is released. The benefits of massage will be spoilt if muscles tense and clench in response to the cold. Ideally, the room should be free from disturbing draughts, yet well-ventilated to allow a healthy circulation of air. Take note of the lighting. Avoid giving a massage in a room with harsh overhead or over-bright lighting. If possible, reduce the light level by turning down the dimmer switch or use only lamps or wall lighting. Shaded, natural light is preferable, or the gentle glow of a candle can add a special touch to the atmosphere.

Choose a suitable chair

The type of chair you use is very important to achieve the most effective massage. You will need one that is fairly upright, preferably without arms. Most kitchen chairs are ideal for the purpose, so long as they do not creak, squeak or wobble. The back of the chair should be low enough to allow you to reach your partner's upper back and shoulders. You must be able to massage without tensing, twisting or straining your back. Your partner should be able to sit comfortably with his or her feet resting firmly on the ground. It is a good idea to experiment with different chairs, using cushions if necessary, to find one that is exactly the right height for you both.

Mood music

Select background music with care. People who spend most of the day in a noisy work or home environment may prefer silence – so always offer the option of quiet. If you decide to play soothing music, choose a piece that you both enjoy. Most good music shops have a selection of tapes and CDs specially composed for massage and relaxation, often featuring natural sounds.

On a warm sunny day, offer your massage partner the ultimate treat of an alfresco massage under the shade of a tree. Or wait until a warm evening, when the stars will add a romantic touch. Take some specially blended oil on holiday and offer an outdoor head massage in a scenic location.

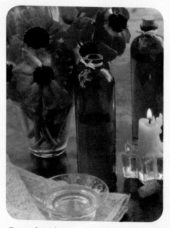

Create the right atmosphere in order to experience the ultimate head massage.

Comfortable clothes

Dress for comfort and practicality. You need to be able to move freely, so choose something loose-fitting, short-sleeved – and washable. Some oils can stain so, if you're concerned about your clothes, drape a towel over your chest or wear an apron and wash it immediately afterward. Always wear freshly laundered clothes, as the stale odour of food or smoke can be most unpleasant. Fresh breath is important too – it is remarkable how the smell of foods, cigarette smoke and coffee can linger. Wear your hair tied back from your face, both for hygiene and practical purposes. Remove your wristwatch and any bracelets, dangling earrings, long necklaces or rings that could interfere with the smooth flow of the massage. Wear low-heeled shoes or go barefoot – if your feet feel comfortable you will be more relaxed.

Avoid distractions

Turn off the television, shut out the sound of traffic, switch on the answerphone and hang a "do not disturb" notice on the door. Check that children and pets are settled for at least half an hour. A valuable feature of Indian head massage is that it allows space in a busy life for some complete "me" time. It gives your massage partner the chance to enjoy the comforting, stress-relieving sensation of being nurtured. Also if you are worried about being disturbed, you will probably find it more difficult to concentrate on the massage.

When head massage is to be avoided

Like all forms of massage, Indian head massage is generally considered a safe, non-invasive therapy. However, there are a few occasions when it can actually cause more harm than good, so do check that your massage partner is not suffering from any conditions, known as contraindications, that could be aggravated by massage.

If you have any doubts – do not give a massage. Trust your intuition and postpone the massage until you have taken professional advice or are certain the condition has cleared up completely.

Points to watch

Never give a massage if your massage partner has any of the following conditions.

- Any recent injuries involving the head, neck, shoulders or limbs, including sprains, strains, fractures and whiplash. Massage to the area could make the injury worse and would also be extremely painful. Wait until you are confident that the injury has healed.

CHECKLIST

Contraindications

- Fever.
- Swellings or inflammation.
- Severe bruising in the massage area.
- High or low blood pressure.
- Skin disorders.
- Scalp infections.
- Arthritis of the upper spine.
- Osteoporosis.
- Diabetes.
- Severe asthma.
- Epilepsy.
- Disorders of the nervous system.
- Protruding veins.
- Recent haemorrhage (bleeding).
- History of thrombosis or embolism.
- Recent head or neck injury.
- Recent surgery involving the head or neck.
- Any potentially fatal condition, such as cancer.

- A history of thrombosis (blood clots in an artery or vein) or embolism (blockage in an artery). Massage may encourage a clot or fragment to break away and enter the bloodstream, where it may become lodged and block the flow of blood to a vital organ.

- Any skin disorders or scalp infections, including weeping eczema, acne, psoriasis and head lice, as massage could irritate and/or spread the condition.

- Recent surgery. Massage might delay the healing of recently formed scar tissue.

- Any potentially fatal condition such as cancer. Although a trained masseur can often help relieve pain and induce relaxation in someone who has contracted cancer, there is a risk of making the condition worse. Try gentle stroking instead.

- Disorders of the nervous system, such as multiple sclerosis, which could be exacerbated by the stimulating effect of massage.

- Osteoporosis. This is a condition, usually associated with the ageing process, in which bones lose their density and become weak and brittle. Strong pressure on fragile bones could cause a fracture.

- A migraine attack. Although Indian head massage can help relieve recurrent migraines, massage during an attack could make the symptoms worse.

Do not massage anyone who is under the influence of alcohol or drugs. It is impossible to know what reaction to expect in these circumstances, so do not take the risk.

Doctor's advice

Seek advice and consent from an appropriate medical practitioner if any of the following situations apply to your massage partner.

- Being prescribed medication, especially strong or long-term drugs, being under medical supervision, or receiving complementary therapies.

- A chronic (on-going) medical condition, such as diabetes, epilepsy, severe asthma, serious heart problems, oedema (fluid retention leading to tissue swelling) or acute back pain.

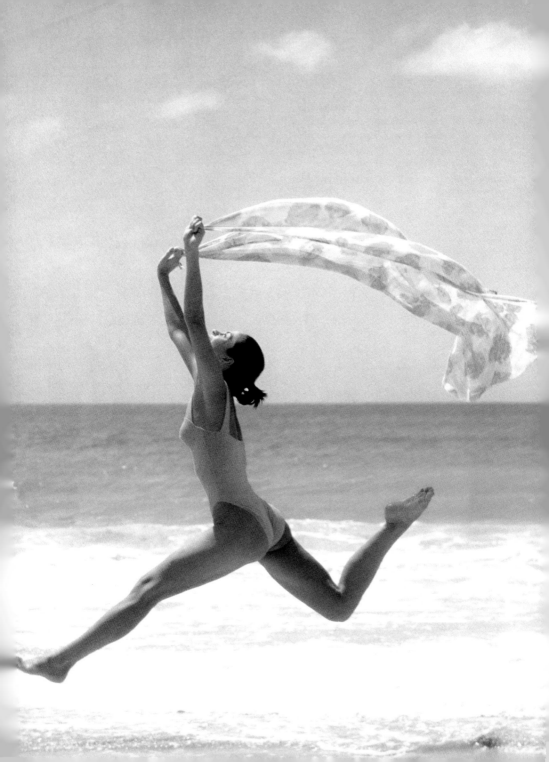

- High or low blood pressure, as massage can cause fluctuations in blood pressure levels.

- Pregnancy. Take particular care during the first three months, when the risk of foetal disorders and miscarriage are greatest. Keep strokes light and gentle. Check that your massage partner has not developed a medical condition such as high blood pressure or gestational diabetes, which are relatively common in pregnancy. Do not use pure essential oils during pregnancy and breastfeeding.

Look out for:

- Fever. Massage is not usually recommended for anyone with a temperature over 37.5°C (99.4°F). A high temperature generally indicates that the body is bringing its defence mechanisms into action to deal with an infection of some kind. Massage increases the body temperature and so might interfere with this natural healing process.

- Swollen, inflamed, bruised, tender or sore muscles, joints or areas of skin. Never massage over swollen lymph nodes. Avoid the affected part or postpone the massage, especially if the cause of the problem is not known, as you may cause further damage.

- Warts, skin tags, moles, boils, bruises, cuts and abrasions, broken skin, blisters, sensitive or protruding veins, areas of sunburn, bites or stings and unexplained lumps. In some cases, you may be able to cover the site with a small plaster. Work very carefully to avoid massaging directly over the area.

Look after your own health

When giving an Indian head massage, you are in such close contact with your massage partner that infectious or contagious conditions could easily be passed on. Be wary of massaging anyone who has a skin and scalp infection or is feeling generally unwell or nauseous. Cover any cuts or abrasions on your own hands to reduce the risk of cross-infection. Postpone the massage if you are feeling below par. You need to reserve your energy for the sake of your own health.

Pre-massage advice

- Ask your massage partner to wait at least an hour after eating a meal or exercising before having the massage, and advise him to avoid stimulants such as tea and coffee immediately before the massage.

- Check any possible adverse reactions or allergies to individual carrier or essential oils. Read all safety guidelines carefully. You must be completely confident that the oils you use have no potentially harmful effects.

- Do not use essential oils on babies, children or elderly people.

CASE STUDY

A good night's sleep

Peter, 60, was persuaded to try Indian head massage by his wife, Moira, because he was sleeping badly and felt permanently tired. "I didn't want to take sleeping tablets," he explained, "but I was becoming desperate – and so was Moira. I was getting forgetful and irritable in the day, then at night I would toss and turn and keep her awake. I was prepared to try anything. Much to my embarrassment, I fell fast asleep during the first head massage. I don't really remember much. I felt quite weird when I woke up – not with it at all. I kept muddling up my words. But I sat still for a little while and soon came round. I almost floated home, I felt so light and relaxed.

"I slept really well that night. It was a lovely surprise to wake up, look at the clock and realise that it was morning. I didn't sleep quite so well on the following nights, but then after my second massage, I had another good night's night. Over a few months of regular Indian head massage and full body massage my sleep patterns have gradually changed for the better. I still get the odd night of wakefulness but generally I get about six or seven hours. I have far more energy in the day – and I'm sure my memory has got better."

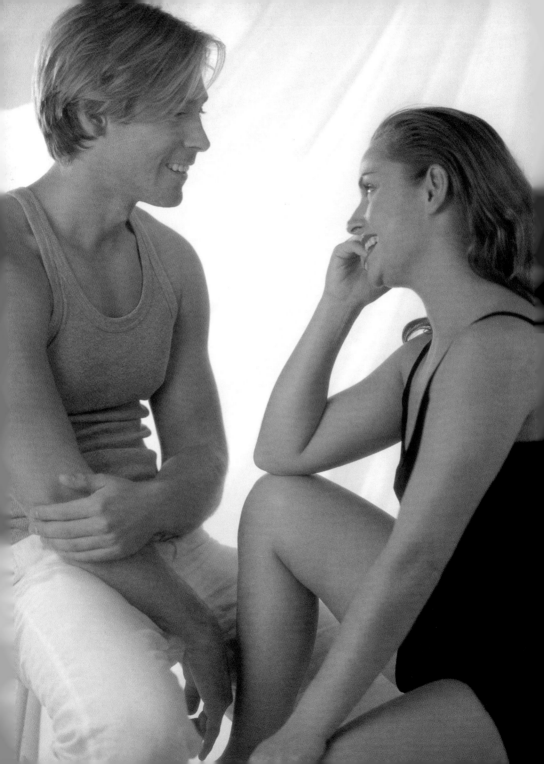

CHAPTER SIX

THE FULL WORKS

A N INDIAN HEAD MASSAGE involves varying combinations of gentle, soothing and brisk, stimulating movements to suit the mood, needs and preferences of the recipient. The following routine takes around 20–30 minutes from start to finish but can be readily adapted by spending longer on favourite strokes, omitting others, or adding some of the movements featured in the other step-by-step sequences, in chapters 7, 8 and 9. A natural vegetable carrier oil – with the addition of a pure essential oil if you wish – acts as a wonderfully nourishing lubricant, but it is possible to perform the massage without oil by doing it through light clothing.

Things you will need

- Upright chair with a low back.
- 10ml of suitable oil in a small bowl (see chapter 3).
- Large towel.
- Small towel draped over a chair back.
- Paper towels to wipe your hands and absorb any spillage.
- Soft background music (optional).
- Clock (helpful to keep an eye on the time).
- Apron (optional).

Things to do

- Dress in comfortable, washable clothes.
- Reduce the lighting.
- Check that the room is warm and free from draughts.
- Switch on the answerphone or unplug the phone. Make sure that you are not likely to be disturbed for the next half an hour or so.
- Remove any jewellery that may interfere with the massage.
- Wash your hands. Ensure your nails are short, smooth, clean and free from nail polish. Cover any cuts or abrasions with a plaster.
- Warm your hands; shake them from the wrists to release any tension.
- Breathe slowly and deeply, concentrating your thoughts on the massage you are about to give. Rehearse the different moves in your mind.
- Adopt a calm, centred approach (see page 62).

Before you begin

Never give a massage without first having a preliminary discussion with your massage partner. Most importantly, check that there are no contraindications that would make it inadvisable to continue (see page 65). Ask about past or current medical problems – particularly accidents, injuries or serious illnesses. Look at the condition of your partner's hair and skin and pick up clues about her general health and well-being. This is also an opportunity to ask questions that will help you to adapt the massage to suit your partner's needs and wishes. Find out if there are any areas that require special attention and ask how she hopes to feel afterward. Has she had an Indian head massage before? If so, ask if she experienced any adverse reactions (see page 110), were there any movements she liked or disliked and does she have any suggestions of her own.

It might seem tempting to launch straight into a massage, but it is worthwhile spending some time reading through the preliminary steps described in this chapter until you are familiar with them, so you do not have to keep stopping to refer to them. You can rehearse the moves quite easily while sitting in a chair by practising on your own thigh and bended knee.

Let your partner know what to expect

The thought of having your head touched in such an intimate way can seem rather daunting. Give your partner the chance to ask questions. Explain about the sequence of movements. Give a brief summary of the benefits and possible reactions (page 110). These are different for everyone and can vary every time.

Explain that comfort is an integral part of the relaxation process. Make it perfectly clear to your massage partner that she should tell you at once if anything about the massage feels painful or unpleasant. You can easily stop and then continue with another movement. Above all, explain that this is her time to relax, shut off from the outside world and thoroughly enjoy being pampered.

CHECKLIST

Advice for your partner

- Remove any make-up, if possible, to ensure optimum benefits from the oil.
- Remove earrings and necklace.
- Remove spectacles or contact lenses.
- Brush through her hair to avoid pulling and tangling.
- Tie up long hair with a clip, head-band or similar accessory.
- Adjust clothing. Your massage partner need not disrobe for a dry massage – a T-shirt or similar light clothing is suitable. For an oily massage, your massage partner should take off her upper clothing and adjust her bra straps to leave her shoulders bare. Wrap a large towel around her chest – warm it on a radiator first for extra comfort.

✿ Massage sequence

✿ Try not to rush any of these movements. A gentle, unhurried pace will contribute greatly to the efficacy of the massage.

Deep breathing

During this deep breathing sequence, you may like to suggest that your partner imagines breathing in peace and tranquillity and expelling any doubts, fears or frustrations. You can do the same. This is also an ideal opportunity to guide your partner through a relaxation exercise (see page 60) if you feel it is appropriate.

1 Place a hand on each shoulder, with your fingers resting on the upper arm facing downward. Turn your body so that your right hip is pushed into your partner's back.

2 Pull her shoulders gently back toward you. As her shoulders move, ask your partner to take a deep breath through her nose. Hold for a couple of seconds. Ask her to breathe out slowly through her mouth as you gradually release the shoulders, pushing them gently back into place. Take longer on the out-breath than the in-breath.

3 Repeat the move very slowly and deliberately at least three times. It helps to talk through the movement so that your partner knows what is expected. "As I take your shoulders back, breathe in deeply and slowly... hold... now, as I release your shoulders, breathe out, long and slow . . . "

Making contact

Resting your hands on your massage partner's head provides a reassuring, comforting moment of contact. It helps make your partner feel secure and creates an awareness of the touch of your hands on his head. This preliminary hold is a very important part of the massage as it helps to establish a bond that allows you both to relax, centre and focus on the massage. Your partner will appreciate the lovely sense of calm that it brings.

With your massage partner seated in a chair, legs uncrossed and feet flat on the floor, gently rest your hands on either side of his head, with your fingers facing toward the crown. Stay still and quiet. Hold for a minute and release very gradually.

CAUTIONS ✿ **Be careful not to press down too firmly on the head as too much pressure can hurt the neck.**

Restful darkness

This helps relax the muscles at the back of the eyes, which can often get strained as a result of long periods spent reading, and doing other close-up work, or driving, especially in poor visibility. Try it yourself when your eyes feel tired; it is very relaxing to be in total darkness.

1 Ask your partner to close her eyes. Hold the palms of your hands over her eyes with the fingers of one hand slightly overlapping those on the other hand, thumbs facing upward.

2 Press very gently so that she is in complete darkness but does not feel restricted. Hold for thirty seconds.

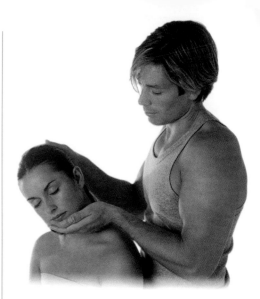

1 Place one hand under your partner's chin for support. Place the other at the back of her head, just below the crown. Gently roll her head in a semi-circle, first to one side, then to the front and around to the other side. Do not roll the head backward as this places unnecessary stress on the neck muscles. Ask your partner to let you support the weight of her head so that you are directing the action.

2 Retrace the line of the arc going in the other direction. Do this movement at least three times, concentrating on detecting any stiffness and tightness. Gently return the head to the upright position and take your hands away slowly.

CAUTIONS ✍ **Keep the head well-supported throughout. Do not press on the throat, as this can be very painful and may restrict breathing.**

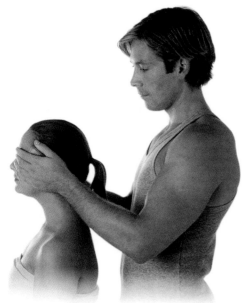

CAUTIONS ✍ **Do check that your partner is not claustrophobic or fearful of darkness before applying this action.**

✍ Apply each stroke with care and love to make your partner feel comforted, reassured and secure.

Head roll

This is a relaxing move that should be carried out very gently as the neck is such a delicate part of the body. Do not force the move. You may find it is quite difficult for your partner to let go at first, but with your reassurance and encouragement she will find that it is a wonderful feeling to allow someone else to support the heaviness of the head. The movement should come from your partner's neck so that only the head moves, not the whole body.

Stroking on the oil

This sequence uses long, confident movements that help soothe and relax your partner.

1 Pour some warm oil into the palm of one of your hands. Some people love to have their hair saturated in oil, whereas others prefer just a little. You can easily top it up during the massage, if you find your partner has very dry skin or long hair.

2 Rub your hands together so that the palms of your hands and fingers are warm and well covered in oil. Explain quietly to your partner that you are now going to stroke the oil into her scalp. This ensures that the feel of oil on her head does not come as a surprise.

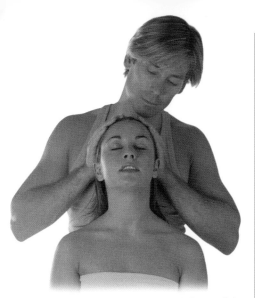

These movements spread the oil and relax and soften the area ready for massage.

Continue with the same flowing movements as before to cover your partner's upper back and upper arms. Use the whole of the palms of both hands and the fleshy pads of the fingers. Start with a very light pressure and gradually make it a little firmer. Keep your hands soft and pliable. The movements are long and slow with a gentle curve.

CAUTIONS Long hair should be tied up or pushed to one side so that it does not get in the way.

Keep breathing slowly and deeply. You will need a good supply of oxygen to help maintain your energy levels. Giving an Indian head massage can be more tiring than you might think. If you find yourself losing concentration, make an effort to think about the strokes.

3 Place both hands on your partner's head, with fingers pointing forward and just touching the start of the hairline. Stroke over the top of the head, using the flat of both hands and the fleshy pads of the fingers to brush against the scalp, and continue along the top of the shoulders. Keep the strokes slow, smooth and flowing. Repeat until you have applied oil to the whole of the scalp.

Maintain as much contact as possible. It can be very disconcerting for your partner if you jerk your hands away suddenly at the end of a move. Gradually decrease the pressure and let your hands float slowly away from her skin.

Thumb fans

This movement works on the powerful kite-shaped trapezius muscle, where many people store a great deal of tension. As you move your thumbs, you will start to feel some movement of the muscle fibres beneath and sense any tightness starting to ease. Your partner may feel some tenderness.

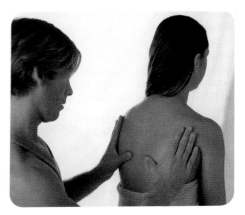

1 Place your hands flat on your partner's back, on either side of the spine, so that the heels of your hands rest just below the bottom of the shoulder-blades, or scapulas. Keep your fingers slightly outstretched and resting lightly on the skin.

2 Press fairly firmly with the sides of your thumb pads and, with one long sweeping fan-like movement, push them upward to the base of the neck and across the top of the shoulders. Your thumbs should stay in contact with the skin as you sweep them up to form a curved T-shape. Maintain a firm, even pressure throughout the stroke.

Warming up

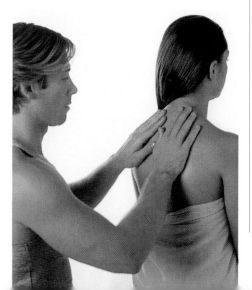

3 Continue until you have covered the whole of the trapezius. This is a deep effleurage movement that helps boost the blood flow to the area and warms and softens the underlying muscle tissues. Work this area for at least a couple of minutes.

CAUTIONS 🖐 **While working with your thumbs, keep your fingers relaxed so that you do not grasp your partner's shoulders too tightly.**

🖐 *Never work directly over the spine, as this protects the spinal cord and contains a vast number of individual nerves linking the brain to all parts of the body.*

Thumb kneading

This sequence involves a petrissage movement that flattens and broadens the muscle tissues, helping to disperse any nodules of tension. It also helps squeeze out any excess lymph and encourages a healthy flow of nourishing blood to feed the muscle fibres and improve the condition of the tissues. Pay special attention to the upper trapezius (feel for the soft tissue that runs along the top of the shoulder) which tends to get very tight. You can also knead this area with the pads of your fingers or the palms of your hands.

1 With your hands held in the same position as before, make deep, circular movements with your thumb pads over the whole of the trapezius muscle. Keep your fingers relaxed as you work with the thumbs. Rotate the skin firmly against the underlying tissues so that you can feel the muscle fibres moving, stretching and loosening beneath your firm touch. Press, lift, squeeze and release the flesh in a rhythmic, kneading action. Stand firmly on two feet and lean into the movement, using your body weight to

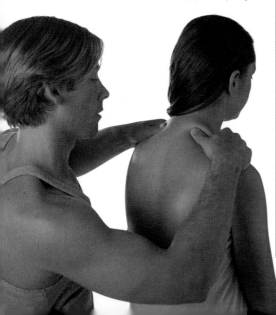

gradually increase the pressure on the upward move and decrease on the downward part of each circle.

2 Work upward with a smooth, continuous action so that your hands do not leave your partner's back and shoulder area. Work the area for around five to seven minutes.

CAUTIONS 🖐 **Be careful not to press too hard or too suddenly and keep the movement flowing. Sudden, jerky actions will make your massage partner even more tense. Watch out for tell-tale body language or ask your partner if the level of pressure is bearable.**

Shoulder sweeping

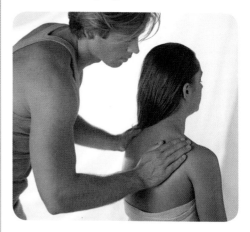

This is a soothing, calming movement that is useful to include at any time during the massage and helps soothe any slight discomfort caused by the previous movement. Deep massage to the trapezius may cause some discomfort but this is usually described as "therapeutic" or "positive" and can bring a great sense of relief. However, too much work on tight muscles can cause the fibres to contract even more and may cause bruising. If your partner is particularly tense around her upper back and shoulders, take it in stages. Repeat the warming up, thumb fans, thumb kneading and shoulder sweeping movements two or three times a week until the tension has cleared.

1 Place your left hand on your massage partner's left shoulder for support. Place the palm of your right hand on the right shoulder-blade, fingers splayed and pointing toward the upper arms.

2 Push the whole of the flat of your hand upward in slow, generous, circular movements, sweeping across the top of the shoulder and tracing the outline of the shoulder-blade. Make sure the flat of your hand is in contact with the skin at all times. Keep your wrist flexible and mould your hand to the shape of your massage partner's back.

3 Use your body weight to increase the depth of pressure on the upward movement and decrease as you slide your hand downward. You can move your hand in a clockwise or anticlockwise direction, whichever feels most comfortable. Repeat at least four times. Now repeat the sequence on the other side, this time with your right hand on your massage partner's right shoulder.

Ironing the shoulders

This is another movement that can be introduced into your massage at any time. It is surprisingly pleasurable for your massage partner, often creating a tingling sensation throughout the whole body. The sliding action helps lower hunched-up shoulders, relaxes the deltoid muscles at the top of the arms and drains toxins down to the lymph nodes in the elbow, for elimination from the body.

1 Place both hands near the base of your partner's neck. Using the outer edges of your hands, "iron" along the top of the shoulders to the upper arm. Press quite firmly, keeping the sides of your hands in contact with the skin. Maintain the same level of pressure throughout the movement.

2 As you reach the top of the upper arms, change the position of your hands, without losing contact with the skin, so that the

flat of the hands sweep downward in a firm, flowing effleurage movement toward the elbows. Do this at least three times, ensuring that the whole of the upper arms have been covered.

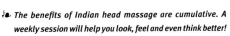

The benefits of Indian head massage are cumulative. A weekly session will help you look, feel and even think better!

Easing a stiff neck

These movements help relax the tension that often builds up in the neck, so easing stiffness and pain and aiding neck mobility.

1 Place one hand on your partner's forehead. Ask her to drop her head forward so that you can support its weight and her neck is easily accessible for massage.

2 With the pads of your fingers or the palm of the other hand, make gentle, circular stroking movements with a very light pressure up the back of the neck to the base of the skull and along the bony ridge, known as the occiput, to the ears. Repeat three or four times to warm the area ready for deeper massage.

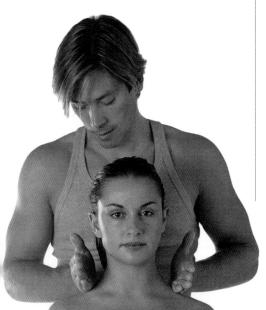

Relaxing scalp tension

Massaging around the base of the skull can help stretch and soften constricted muscle fibres, boost the flow of blood and release any buildup of toxins, so easing tension headaches, which often start around this area. You may find that your massage partner's scalp is very tight, if she is under a lot of stress. As she relaxes, you should start to feel the scalp loosening and moving more easily.

1 With one hand supporting the head and your other hand in the same V shape position as in the previous sequence, make small static frictions with the pads of your thumbs and fingers along both sides of the bony ridge. Starting from the top of the spine, work out toward the ears. Press the scalp firmly along the ridge of the bone, hold for a couple of seconds, then release. Lift and repeat a little further along until the whole occiput has been covered.

2 Follow the same path, this time making small circular friction movements. Repeat on the same spot for three circles, then lift your hand and move to the next spot. Now do these two movements again, this time using the other hand to support the head.

CAUTIONS 🖐 **When working on the occiput you should massage the scalp against the bone and avoid pressing on the fleshy area beneath the bone, as this may cause nausea.**

🖐 *Try not to catch your massage partner's hair when massaging her scalp. If you feel that you may be pulling it, lift your hands away and start again.*

3 Form a V between the thumb and first finger and lightly clasp the base of your massage partner's neck. Stand firmly on both feet, ensuring that her head is well supported with one hand at all times. Place your thumb on the fleshy area on one side of the bony cervical vertebrae and the pads of one or two fingers on the other side.

4 Starting at the base of the neck, work upward with a gentle kneading action. Lift, squeeze and release the muscles in a rhythmic, rotating movement.

5 Massage up to the bony ridge at the base of the skull, then give the muscles a slight stretch, without moving the head.

6 Repeat the movement, using the other hand over the same area – you will find that it feels completely different with each hand. It is best to work with your non-dominant hand first.

7 Finish with some soothing stroking up the neck.

CAUTIONS 🖐 **The neck area can be very tender, so ask your partner to tell you how much pressure feels comfortable.**

🖐 *Never press hard on the neck. Stop if your partner experiences any pain, dizziness or discomfort.*

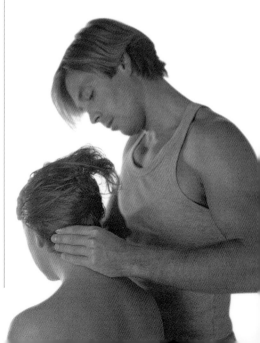

Brisk rubbing

Brisk rubbing continues the benefits of the previous kneading technique by stimulating the blood and lymph circulation.

1 With the head still firmly supported in one hand, as before, use the fleshy pads of two or three fingers to rub along one side of the occiput from the top of the neck to behind the ear. Briskly rub along the bone backward and forward in a short, rapid sawing action. If you massage in a circular motion you will find that the hair tends to get rather matted.

2 Change hands and repeat on the other side. Repeat three times. Try this rubbing movement with the heel or side of your hand.

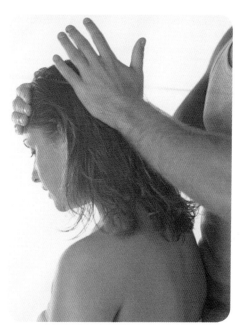

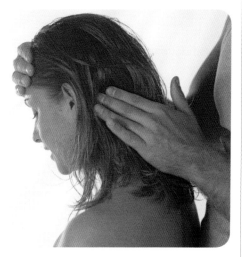

CAUTIONS 🖐 Keep your hand moving swiftly. Do not stay in the same place for long.

🖐 Be aware of your posture. Stand with your feet shoulder-width apart to maintain a good balance. Keep your back straight and your shoulders relaxed so you are in a comfortable position to give an effective massage without straining your back. Move around your partner's chair so that you do not need to strain to reach. Kneel on the floor or bend your knees if you need to lower yourself for a particular move.

Warming the scalp

In this technique, the pressure should be fairly firm so you are working on the scalp to stimulate the local blood circulation and warm the area. Your massage partner's hair will look a real mess afterwards – but with regular massage it will be far more healthy!

1 Keep your partner's head well-supported with one hand, as before, and continue the brisk rubbing, moving up from the occiput to the crown. Keep your wrists fairly flexible and use the palm or heel of your hand in a rapid, waving action.

2 When you reach the crown, lift your hand and start again, a little further around the back of the head. Repeat several times so that the whole of the back of the head has been covered.

CAUTIONS 🖐 Maintain a firm support for the head so that you can push against your supporting hand to increase the pressure without causing discomfort in your partner's neck. Keep your hands moving over the scalp – do not work over the same spot for any length of time.

"Shampooing" the scalp

This movement usually comes quite naturally as most of us have experienced it at the hairdresser's. Indeed, many people comment that the best thing about going to a hair salon is having the shampoo massaged into their head. It is a friction movement that stimulates the blood and lymph circulation in the area and warms and loosens the scalp. As the scalp starts to move more freely, the tension is eased, bringing a great sense of well-being. "Shampooing" just behind the ears feels lovely. This movement takes practice, so try it on yourself to improve the circulation in your own scalp.

1 Place your hands on either side of the scalp, with fingers well spread out so that your little fingers are resting on your partner's temples and your thumbs are at the back of her head.

2 With your hands held in this position, place your fingers in a wide claw-like pose and use the fleshy pads of your fingers and thumbs to make small anticlockwise movements all over the scalp. Keep your fingers fairly rigid so that you can feel the scalp moving beneath them. The action is slow and deliberate with a firm, even pressure. Repeat three times so that the entire scalp is covered.

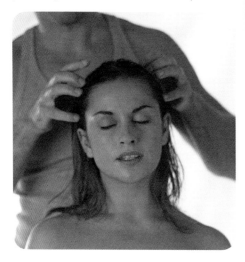

CAUTIONS Ensure that your partner's head is held firmly between your two hands and is well supported. If you find it difficult to "shampoo" with both hands, place one on your partner's brow to support her head and massage with the other. Change hands as necessary.

Finger tapping

The following action is rhythmical but there is no need for your fingers to tap in any particular order. It is rather like playing the piano or drumming your fingers on the table to show impatience. It is an energizing, revitalizing action, a gentle form of tapotement that helps stimulate the blood circulation in the scalp.

With the hands held in the same position as before, tap the pads of your fingers alternately all over your partner's scalp and the back of the neck. Keep your fingers fairly flexible so you can tap the head quickly, energetically and firmly without being too heavy handed. Your fingers should bounce back up again as soon as they land.

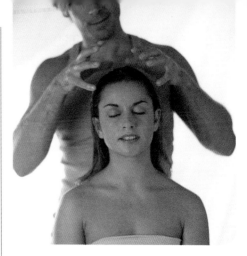

Hair smoothing

This is a soothing, relaxing movement that contrasts well with the previous brisker strokes and helps drain any excess blood or lymph from the scalp. It provides a good opportunity to put your partner's hair back in place.

Rest both hands lightly on your massage partner's head, with fingers facing forward. Using alternate hands, stroke from the top of your partner's head right down to her shoulders in a flowing, gently overlapping motion. As one hand finishes, the other hand starts so that continuity is maintained. Keep your fingers and hands soft and moulded to the contours of your partner's head, neck and shoulders.

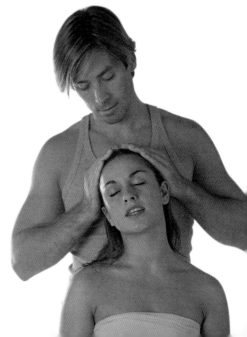

✆ Facial massage

You are now going to massage your partner's face. But before you begin, there are some important points to consider. Firstly, check that your partner's neck is not strained. The head can become surprisingly floppy during a facial massage. If her head is allowed to fall back too far, it not only causes discomfort, but can also restrict breathing, leading to feelings of panic. Your partner's head should feel secure and supported throughout so that she can relax completely and gain maximum benefits from the massage.

Stand close to her back and use a rolled up towel to support her neck so that her head is resting firmly against your chest. Maintain this stance throughout. This position is also useful for a woman giving a massage who may feel slightly inhibited about having a man resting his head against her chest. Keep a rolled up towel ready so that you do not disturb the flow of the massage.

You should always keep your massage partner warm and cosy. Wrap a towel around her shoulders so that she does not get chilly while you are working on her face. Drape a towel over the back of the chair for this purpose. You can also use the towel to dab off any excess oil on your partner's back or shoulders.

Check the amount of oil on your hands and fingers. There should be just enough oil to provide light lubrication for a smooth massage without dragging the skin. Wipe off any excess. Look for any stray hairs that may be on your hands and remove them before you massage the delicate skin on the face.

Forehead stroking

This is a caring, soothing stroke that is wonderfully relaxing. Habitual frowning or worried expressions can cause these muscles to constrict, which leads to furrowed brows, tension headaches and eye strain. Gentle stroking helps ease the tension from these overworked muscles and smoothes away fine tension lines.

1 Place your hands on your partner's forehead so that your fingers overlap slightly, with the thumbs pointing upward. Using the flat of three fingers, stroke away from the centre of the forehead toward the temples.

2 Start just above the eyebrows and repeat a little higher, gradually moving up to the hairline. Your hands work in alternate finger-over-finger strokes so that it feels like one continuous movement. Repeat around six times until the whole of the forehead has been covered. Keep the movement very slow, with a light, even pressure. Your hands should be soft and gently moulded to the shape of the brow.

✆ *Keep the pressure on the face very light. Do not drag the skin. If necessary, add a little more oil.*

Temple circles

The temples are another tension hot-spot where constricted muscles are a common cause of headaches and eye strain. Massage helps boost the circulation of blood and lymph and relaxes the temporalis muscles, often within a matter of minutes. You can also try this movement using the heels of your hands. This is a very slow and controlled movement using a fairly firm pressure – so do not be tempted to speed it up.

Place your hands over your massage partner's temples. Using the pads of two fingers, massage the temples with small, clockwise or anticlockwise movements. Avoid digging in with your fingertips. Keep your fingers on the same spot – it is the skin that moves as you make the rotations. Make around twelve circles.

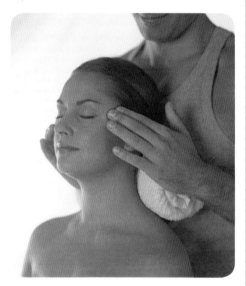

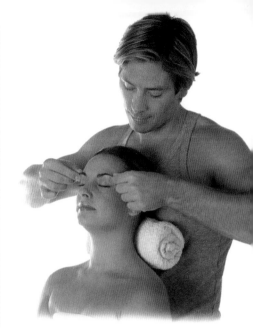

1 Gently hold your partner's eyebrows between the pads of your thumbs and index fingers. Gently squeeze, pressing fairly firmly against the bone. Hold for a couple of seconds and release. Start at the bridge of your partner's nose and work out toward the temples.

2 Lift and move to the next spot. Repeat until the whole of the eyebrows have been covered. Return to the starting position. Repeat three times. Finish with a few gliding strokes along the eyebrows, smoothing the hairs back into position.

CAUTIONS ✍ **Do not apply pressure if your partner's sinuses are swollen or painful.**

✍ *When massaging near the eyes, be careful not to allow any oil to seep into your partner's eyes. If it does, wash with cold water immediately.*

CAUTIONS ✍ **It is important to find the right area of the temple. Feel for the shallow depression surrounded by a bony ridge at the corner of your partner's eyes. Work on this small area of soft tissue.**

✍ *Do not be concerned if you partner falls asleep – keep going. When someone has trouble getting to sleep, an Indian head massage in the late evening can work wonders.*

Eyebrow squeeze

This sequence helps relieve the tension that often builds up in the muscles and helps ease any congestion in the sinus passages around the eyes. The area may be a little tender but these movements are surprisingly calming.

Clearing sinus congestion

In this sequence, the compression action of your fingers mimics a pump and helps draw out any lymph in the sinus passages. You may feel some slight puffiness in the area if your partner suffers from congested sinuses. She may even hear or feel some "popping" during this movement. This is an indication that the sinuses are starting to clear.

1 Place the index finger of each hand near the sides of your partner's nostrils. Following the line of the cheekbones (or zygomatic bones), apply small static frictions with the pad on one finger, pushing the flesh firmly up and under the ridge of the bones. Press, hold for a count of a few seconds, release and move to the next spot. Work slowly and precisely, right along to the sides of the face, lessening the pressure as you reach the ears. Return to the starting position and repeat three times.

2 Now make sweeping movements with one finger along the same paths to help direct the excess lymph to the lymph nodes near the ears, where it can be filtered and purified. Repeat these sinus sweeps three times. This is an excellent movement to use on yourself.

Clenching and grinding teeth are common signs of stress that cause these muscles to become over-tight and painful, often leading to headaches and irritability.

1 Place your fingers at each corner of your partner's mouth. Using the pads of your fingers, gently stroke, one hand after the other, outward across her cheeks toward her ears. As one stroke finishes so the other begins, in a flowing action. Repeat three times.

2 Using the pads of two fingers, rub lightly but briskly all around the sides of her mouth and outward to her ears. Always move upward to help tone and lift the muscles. You may also like to apply small, anticlockwise, circular movements around these areas with the pads of two fingers. Finish by repeating the initial stroking action.

CAUTIONS 🌿 **Massaging around the jaw area can be very uncomfortable if your partner is wearing dentures. If possible, remove the dentures. Otherwise use a very gentle touch.**

🍃 *Releasing tension in the facial muscles can have an almost instant effect. Your partner's face will look softer, more relaxed and refreshed.*

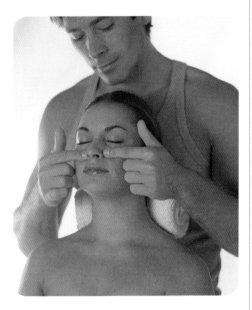

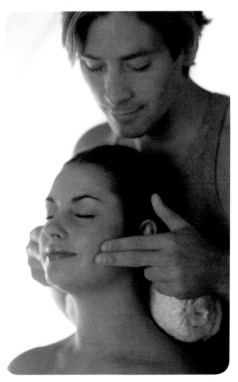

CAUTIONS 🌿 **Miss out this movement if your partner's sinuses are extremely congested or painful.**

🍃 *Lightly rubbing and stroking the ears can have a very pleasurable and sensual effect – so save this for a romantic evening for two. Massage the insides of the ears too.*

Releasing tension along the jaw line

This is a similar movement to the back and forth waving type action performed on the occiput, but your pressure should be light so that your fingers move superficially over the skin. These movements help warm and soften the jaw muscles, especially the powerful masseter muscles.

Facial tapping

This is a soft tapotement movement that stimulates the blood circulation helps firm the facial muscles and gives the skin a radiant glow.

1 Tap the pads of your fingers very gently all over your partner's face and neck in a random but rhythmical fashion. The action is similar to "Finger tapping" (see page 78) but your touch should be much lighter. Do not forget to work under the chin – the jowl area often tends to slacken with age, resulting in a doublechin.

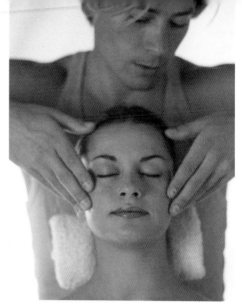

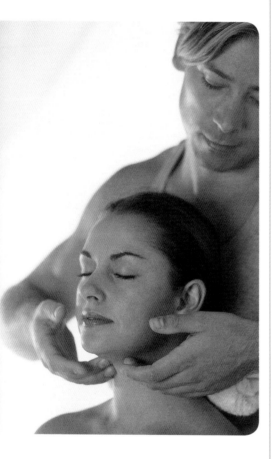

1 With the flat of four fingers, stroke from your partner's neck up the face to the hairline in long, gliding, caressing strokes. Use alternate hands in a smooth, wave-like flowing motion so that as one stroke finishes the other begins. Keep your wrists flexible and your hands moulded to the natural shape of her face.

2 Finish each stroke with a soft, lifting action, as though encouraging the muscles to defy the force of gravity. Do at least ten feather-like strokes so that the whole of her face is covered. Do not miss out the upper lip area and sides of the face.

Repeat restful darkness

By repeating the restful darkness sequence you allow your partner to enjoy the calming effect of total darkness.

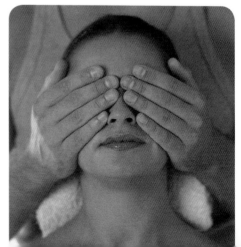

Facial stroking

Follow the previous stimulating movements with gentle stroking. This soothes the many sensory nerve endings in the face and releases mood-enhancing endorphins to promote a sense of inner harmony and serenity.

Final touch

Repeat the first sequence – "Making contact" (see page 71). Maintain this reassuring hold for about half a minute and then gradually release your hands and step back. Stand silently by your massage partner's side for a couple of minutes to allow her to awaken slowly from a state of deep relaxation. She may feel very "spaced out" and need time to gather her thoughts. Suggest that she stays seated while you wash your hands and bring her a glass of water. Advise her to put on a warm cardigan or sweater after the massage. If circumstances permit, wrap her hair in a warm towel and suggest that she rests for at least half an hour before washing off the oil.

Oil will wash out of hair very easily afterward. The trick is to apply a little neat shampoo straight on to the hair. Do not wet the hair first. Rub in the shampoo, rinse in warm water and then wash as normal.

CASE STUDY

Computer-aided tension

Steve, 38, works in a busy architectural practice as a computer-aided design technician. Deadlines tend to be so tight that he often spends all day working at the computer with very few breaks. "When you're working you don't notice how tense your muscles have become," he explained. "It's only when you stop that your body feels stiff and painful. I often used to go home with aching eyes, a sore head and fuddled brain. But it wasn't really enough to bother about; you learn to put up with it. Then, a couple of months ago, a local therapist wrote to the office offering his services in Indian head massage. It seemed like such a good idea

so we decided to find out more.

"I enjoyed the first session so much that I booked in for a weekly head massage. It only takes about 20 minutes and it is done at my desk. Afterward, I feel alert and focused. I seem to be able to get the work done much quicker with a more creative flare. I still spend long hours at the computer but I take more breaks. If I feel a headache brewing I massage my temples, which is very soothing. I enjoy the evenings far more because I don't have so many aches and pains. My children tell me that I am far less grumpy!"

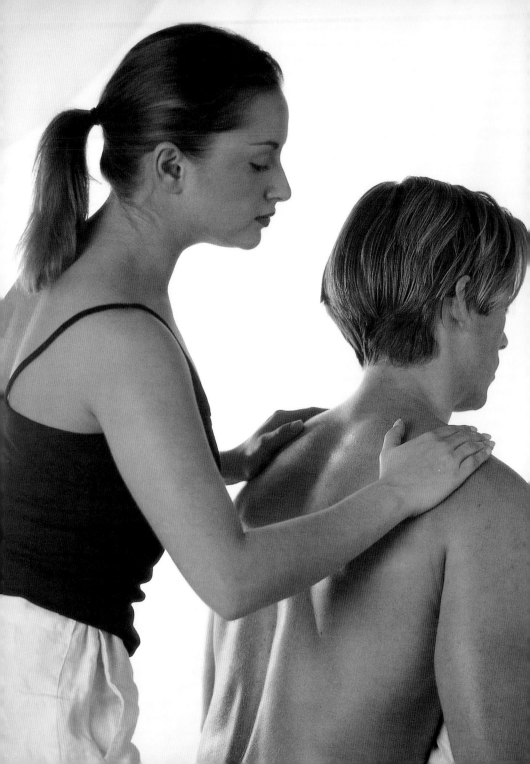

CHAPTER SEVEN

INSTANT ENERGY

ASHORT, BRISK INDIAN HEAD MASSAGE can be amazingly revitalizing. Try this 5–10 minute sequence of stimulating movements to refresh and invigorate weary friends or family members. It is a perfect pick-me-up for those times when energy levels are low but the demands of living are high – such as during a mid-afternoon vitality slump, or in the evening when you have had an exhausting day at work or have spent hours travelling. Your massage partner may find it more comfortable to straddle a chair, preferably leaning against a large cushion or pillow covered with a towel. The use of oil is optional, depending on when and where you give the massage. The movements can be just as effective through light clothing.

Revitalizing breath

When you are tired, you naturally yawn to fill your body with fresh supplies of reviving oxygen. Controlled breathing is a better way to combat lethargy. You and your partner can practise the following breathing technique together. It may help to imagine that you are breathing in energy, vitality and enthusiasm and breathing out tiredness and listlessness.

1 Start your routine by standing near an open window. Ask your partner to stand squarely, with his feet shoulder-width apart and arms hanging loosely by his sides. You should do the same. You should both feel as relaxed and comfortable as possible.

2 You both take in a long, slow breath through the nose. Hold it, while you count to four in your mind, then exhale slowly but strongly through your mouth, so you really empty your lungs. Take your time on the out-breath. This helps expel the stale air in your lungs and encourages you to take in more oxygen on the next in-breath. Repeat at least four times.

Lowering the shoulders

This sequence helps to establish contact and encourages your massage partner to let go of any exhausting tension.

1 Your partner now sits down with his upper back easily accessible for massage. Place your hands on the top of his shoulders. Hold for a few seconds.

2 Gradually use your body weight to apply more pressure so that you are pushing down on his shoulders. Hold for twenty seconds then release. Ask him to exhale as you lean your weight down. Repeat three times.

Wake-up shake

This is a stimulating movement that helps loosen tight muscle at the top of the trapezius. The sequence involves a smooth and rhythmic action. It is not the vigorous back and forth shoulder-shaking action sometimes used in anger.

1 With your hands resting on your partner's shoulders, lightly grasp the upper part of the trapezius muscle (the soft tissue that runs along the top of the shoulders).

2 Gently move the muscle mass on each shoulder backward and forward in an alternate shaking action, one after the other. It is the soft tissue that moves, the shoulders remain fairly still. Do around 10 shakes.

CAUTIONS ✍ **Do not grasp the shoulders too tightly; keep your fingers loose.**

✍ Massage should never cause pain. Be aware of the sounds and movements your massage partner makes. Moans, groans, twitches and faster breathing can all be signs of discomfort. Remind your partner to tell you if anything hurts or causes discomfort.

Stimulating stroking

This invigorating sequence helps apply the oil, brings a fresh supply of oxygenated blood to the area to nourish, warm and revitalize tired muscles, and boosts the lymph circulation. Keep the movements flowing, firm and fairly speedily to stimulate and refresh. If you are using oil, put a little in the palm of one hand and rub your hands together briskly so that they are warm and well lubricated.

1 Make sweeping movements with the whole of the flat of your hands around your partner's shoulders, upper back and upper arms.

2 Place one hand on your partner's left shoulder for support. With the heel of your right hand, rub briskly over his upper back and shoulders, avoiding the spine. Do not be too vigorous over any bony areas. Keep your wrists flexible and rub backward and forward in short, swift movements. Work in all directions, so that you cover the whole of the trapezius muscle, including the top of the shoulders. Repeat, this time with the other hand supporting the right shoulder.

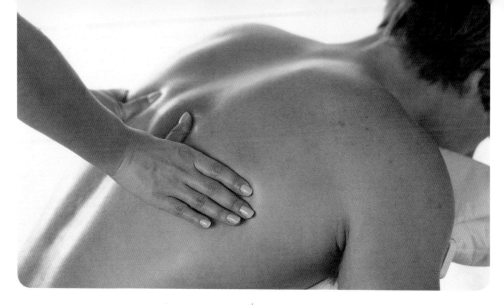

Thumb pressures

This sequence uses a very deep, penetrating friction movement. It can be most effective in relieving muscular tension and stiffness around the shoulder-blades.

1 With your fingers resting lightly on your partner's shoulder-blades, place your thumbs at the base of the shoulder-blades, on either side of the spine. Use the fleshy pads of your thumbs to press firmly in a state of friction. Hold for a couple of seconds and then release.

2 Lift your thumbs and glide up a little. Repeat step 1. Use your body weight to lean into the movement, gradually increasing the pressure. Ask your partner to exhale as you apply pressure and inhale as the pressure is released. Repeat until you have covered the whole of the large trapezius muscle. You may find that your partner's body moves forward as you press firmly.

CAUTIONS 🐾 **If your partner is very tense, these pressures can be painful when applied to a tender spot. If he shows any discomfort, use some gentle, soothing stroking to calm the area.**

🐾 *If you have any doubts about your partner's health or medical condition, do not massage.*

Light hacking on the back

This is very effective for stimulating sensory nerve endings and can be most exhilarating. When you are doing this hacking technique correctly, you will hear a sound similar to the clip-clop of horse's hooves.

1 Hold your hands slightly apart, palms facing each other. Use the little finger side of your hands, known as the ulnar borders, to work alternately in a hacking action (see page 54). Strike the

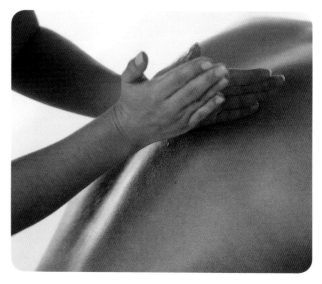

upper back, then release, strike, then release. Keep your wrists flexible and fingers fairly relaxed as you move your forearms up and down. It is a swift, rhythmic action. As soon as each hand touches the skin, it flicks back up again.

2 Hack across the whole area, including the upper trapezius, which runs along the top of the shoulders. Keep moving your hands so you do not overwork any particular spot. Continue for around thirty seconds and then soothe and calm the area with some fairly speedy effleurage strokes.

CAUTIONS ✍ **Avoid massaging over the spine as it contains the vulnerable and highly sensitive spinal cord. Hacking over any bony protrusions can be extremely painful for both you and your massage partner.**

Finger combing

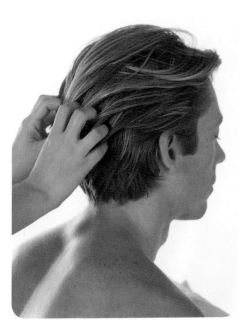

This sequence uses a raking action that creates a completely different sensation to that of using the fleshy pads of your fingers and can often make your partner's scalp tingle. Try it on yourself. It is a useful energizing, circulation-boosting movement.

1 Place both hands in a claw-like position on the top of your partner's head, with your fingers facing forward, just touching the hairline. Keep your fingers fairly widely spread.

2 Use your fingertips to rake back firmly along the scalp, down to the base of the skull. Cover the entire scalp. Your hands can "comb" the hair at the same time or with alternate strokes.

🖐 *Check that your pressure suits your massage partner. Everyone has their own preferences, so adapt to suit.*

Hair tousling

This tousling action stimulates the blood and lymph circulation and helps loosen the muscles in the scalp. This movement can also be performed with one hand, using the other to support the head.

1 With your hands in the same claw-like position as in the previous sequence, use your fingertips to rub firmly and briskly in short random back-and-forth movements all over your partner's scalp. Keep your wrists very flexible and your touch light to medium. Start at the back of the ears and cover the whole head.

2 Keep your hands moving; do not stay in the same place for too long. You may start to feel a lovely, tingling sensation in your fingertips. Your partner's hair should be well and truly ruffled!

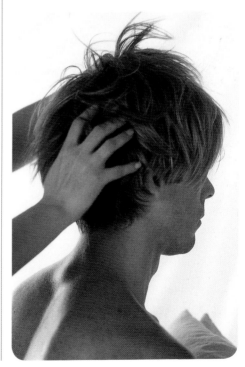

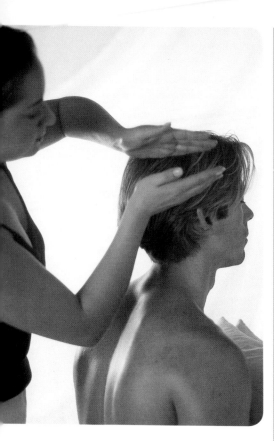

Hair tugging

This sequence is wonderfully revitalizing but be careful not to cause any pain. If your partner appears to flinch, use a lighter touch or move on to the next step. Keep your hands moving so you do not pull the same roots. Hold as much hair as you can.

1 Push your fingers up through your partner's hair and mould the flat of your hands to the shape of his head. Your fingers should be fairly widely spread with large bunches of hair between them. Press the palm of your hand firmly on his scalp around the occiput then grasp the hair roots between your fingers and give it a gentle tug to ease any tension and tiredness. Hold for a few seconds then release.

2 Reposition your hands and repeat the movement three times, until the back of the head has been covered. If your partner has very short hair, you can adapt the technique by clasping the hair roots between your fingers and thumbs, or in a clenched fist with the backs of your fingers against the scalp, and then gently tugging.

CAUTIONS 🐾 **Avoid this movement if your partner has very fine hair.**

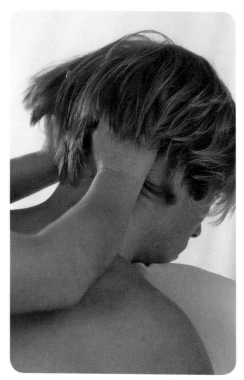

Gentle hacking on the head

Using the same technique as in the "Light hacking on the back" sequence (see page 88), hack very lightly and gently around the sides of your partner's head for about thirty seconds.

CAUTIONS 🐾 **Do not hack over your partner's crown as this can be a very sensitive area and should always be treated with extreme care.**

🐾 *Massage has a powerful influence on sensory nerve endings and can be used to relax or stimulate both mind and body. Energizing strokes are fast and brisk.*

Final flourish

This finishing sequence will leave your partner relaxed and refreshed, ready to continue the day with renewed energy.

1 Repeat the "Finger combing" sequence (see page 89) using first the fingertips and then the soft pads of your fingers to soothe and calm the scalp after the previous invigorating massage movements.

2 Complete the massage by using the flat of your hands to swiftly sweep down your partner's neck and over his shoulders and upper back several times.

3 Allow your massage partner to sit quietly for a few minutes while you wash your hands and bring him a glass of cool, fresh water. This is the ideal time for your partner to enjoy a refreshing shower.

CASE STUDY

Managing a stressful life

John, 46, runs his own painting and decorating business. He spends his spare time renovating an old barn where he plans to live with his wife and their two teenage children. With so many commitments and demands on his energy, life can get stressful at times. So when John heard that Indian head massage could aid relaxation and boost energy levels, he immediately booked in for a course of six sessions – and it has worked, but the results were not immediate. "After the first massage, I felt so exhausted that I went to bed at eight in the evening. The next thing I knew, the alarm was going off. Even after such a good night's sleep, I felt really tired all the next day. I also had a slight, niggling headache. Thankfully, I had been warned that this may happen so I kept sipping

water. I tried to view it as a positive sign that my body was being cleansed of all that alcohol and junk food.

"I am really glad that I booked six weeks of massages in advance – otherwise I might not have gone back. I must admit that I was bit disappointed at the time, I expected to be bursting with health and energy as soon as I walked out of the door. I felt a bit off-colour after my next two massages but it only lasted a few hours. Then after the fourth massage I had no ill effects, and felt bursting with energy. It was incredible. I feel much calmer and less hassled. It has really made me realize that you have got to listen to your body – you cannot keep soldiering on with only a few hours' sleep a night."

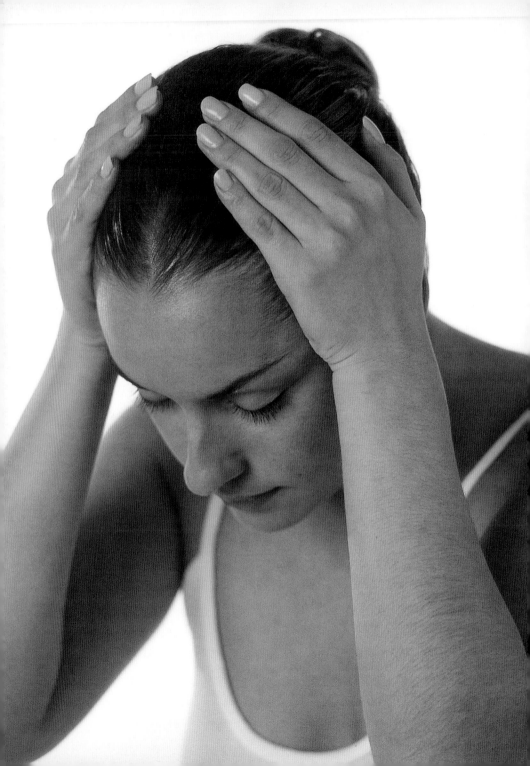

CHAPTER EIGHT

EASE YOUR HEADACHE

W HEN A TENSION HEADACHE strikes you need instant relief. The following five-minute self-massage routine has been devised to ease the pain as soon as it starts, without having to resort to popping painkillers. There is no need to undress or use oil so you can easily perform it wherever you are – at home or at work.

✆ Causes of tension headache

Headaches can cause different degrees of pain, ranging from a dull ache to very severe pain. They have a wide variety of causes, including lack of sleep, stuffy atmosphere, loud noise, changes in the weather, hormonal swings, food intolerances, dehydration, eye strain and poor posture. The most intense form of headache is migraine, which is often accompanied by nausea, dizziness and visual disturbances. However, by far the most common type is the stress or tension headache, which can affect us all at some time or another. Indeed, it has been estimated that the stress-induced kind accounts for four out of every five headaches reported to family doctors.

Tension headaches are usually triggered by tightness in the muscles of the neck, shoulders, scalp and face. This restricts the normal flow of blood and lymph, leading to tenderness and pain, often in localized areas such as the base of the skull, temples, jaws, forehead or sides of the head. Muscular tension is often associated with stress, anxiety, tiredness and long periods spent working at a computer or driving a car. The pain is sometimes described as a "tight band around the head" that gets worse as the day progresses.

It is hard to think straight when your head hurts. It is often tempting just to swallow a painkiller to clear the symptoms so you can carry on with your activities. However, if the underlying cause remains unchecked your tension headaches will keep coming back. Frequent use of painkillers

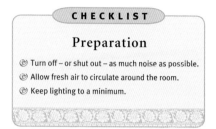

can even cause the very headaches you were trying to alleviate. The key to relieving tension headaches is in relaxation.

🞄 *Most headaches are not a cause for concern. However, you should consult your doctor if the pain is very severe or persistent or the headache is accompanied by fever, vomiting, altered vision, stiff neck or a rash.*

Self-massage for tension relief

A regular relaxation routine (see page 60) helps you to cope better with the stressful situations that often lead to further muscular tension and headaches. Massaging the neck, shoulders, scalp and face can also help by easing the tension in taut muscles – thereby restoring the blood and lymph flow through the tissues, draining the toxins and reducing the pain.

CASE STUDY

Soothing road rage

Jane, 32, has been an insurance sales person for a year, and loves her work. However, it involves long hours and a great deal of time sitting in her car travelling between appointments. After a few months in the job she began to get shooting pains in her shoulders and had almost constant stiffness in her neck. "I was getting really fed up and thinking of changing jobs," she said. "Then a friend recommended Indian head massage and after the first session I realized how tense I had become – both physically and mentally. I'm not a very relaxed person at the best of times, but I was getting very short-tempered – especially with other road-users.

"After just one Indian head massage my neck felt two inches longer and far more mobile, and the constant

nagging thud in my head had cleared. It recurred a few days later but my therapist said it would take a few sessions to clear the problem. She also advised me that Indian head massage doesn't work on its own. I needed to make some lifestyle changes too. She suggested that I take more exercise, correct my posture in the car and try to allow more time between appointments so I am not always rushing. I have learnt to recognize when I'm feeling anxious or certain muscles are beginning to tighten – and I make a real effort to relax. Now I feel happier and more tolerant than ever."

Breathing out tension

Start with a breathing exercise. Stop whatever you are doing. Sit down and close your eyes. Try to close your mind to outside disturbances. Focus on your breathing.

1 Breathe slowly and deeply in through your nose and out through your mouth. On the in-breath concentrate on taking deep, even breaths so that the air flows right down to your abdomen.

2 On the out-breath make a long controlled sigh so that you slowly let out the breath as though exhaling all your tensions. The out-breath should take the same time as or longer than the in-breath. Repeat three times.

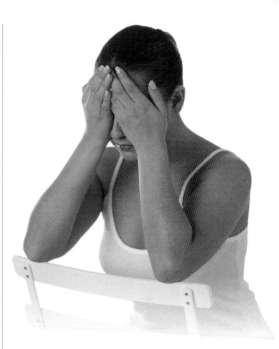

Soothing darkness

Bathing in darkness has such as calming influence that it may be enough to lift a slight headache. Try to switch off from any circling thoughts, think of a colour or concentrate on your breathing.

1 Place your elbows, shoulder-width apart, on a table, chair back or desk in front of you. If you are in a stationary car, rest them on the steering wheel. Lean forward slightly so that your hands support the weight of your head, allowing the release of tension in your neck. Find the most comfortable position.

2 Place your hands over your eyes to create total darkness, enabling the muscles at the back of your eyes to relax. There are many different ways of covering your eyes, so experiment to find which one suits you best. One of the most effective is to place the heels of your hands on your cheekbones, with your palms cupping your eyes, fingers pointing upward. Stay in this position for at least a minute, longer if possible.

Headaches can sometimes be caused by dental problems and poor eyesight, so make an appointment with your optician or dentist if you suffer regular unexplained headaches.

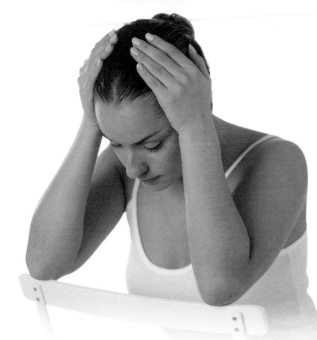

Head hold

The comforting feeling of your hands against your head can help ease you into a state of relaxation.

1 Cradle your head securely between your hands so that the heels of your hands are resting on your temples and your fingers meet at the top of your head. Exert as much pressure with your hands as feels comfortable. Hold for a minute.

2 Move your hands a little further back and repeat this head hold.

Scalp lift

This is a wonderful tension-buster that you can also use with your family and friends. It helps ease out all the tension that is trapped in the thin layer of muscle covering the head.

1 Interlock your fingers and slowly press the palms of your hands inward and upward against your scalp, so that the skin starts to move beneath your fingers.

2 Move to another position and repeat. You can repeat the move as often as you wish.

Keep focusing on your breathing as you massage your scalp. Take deep calming breaths to help relieve any mental and physical tensions.

Scalp de-stressing

This sequence helps loosen the tight and constricted muscles in the neck and is especially soothing if, like many people, you store a lot of tension in this area.

1 Press firmly with the pads of one or two fingers on the soft tissue either side of the cervical vertebrae at the back of your neck. Start at the base and work upward. Hold for a few seconds and then release.

2 Lift your hand and glide on to an adjacent spot. Continue these small static frictions along the bony ridge, or occiput, at the base of the skull, working from the centre and over the arch of the ears to the temples. Start with a fairly light pressure and gradually increase the depth, depending on how you feel. Work along the ridge three times.

3 Repeat the move, making small circular rotations along the occiput. If you wish, you can continue these static or circular frictions up the back of the head and all over the scalp.

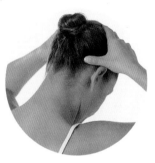

Massaging the temples

You may instinctively rub your temples at the onset of a headache – it is a very effective pain-relieving movement. You will need to locate the soft indentation of both temples. This is often quite difficult to do on yourself, but you will know when you have found the right spot because it feels so good.

Place your hands on your temples. With the heel of your hands or pads of your fingers, make at least ten small circular movements, clockwise or anticlockwise, which-ever feels best. Keep your fingers on the skin and move it against the underlying soft tissue to soften and relax the muscles.

We all hold tension in different places around the head, neck and shoulders. Vary the routine and moves to suit your own personal needs. Massaging your own shoulders with gentle kneading can be very effective.

Soothing a furrowed brow

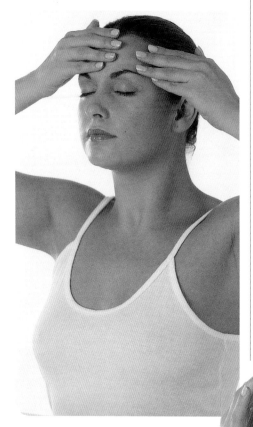

In the following stroking sequence, you will need to use pressure that is firm enough to be effective without making your headache even worse. Keep the movements very, very slow and nurturing.

1 Move your hands up to your forehead. Using the pads of your fingers in a soft, flowing movement, gently stroke away the tension from your forehead.

2 Experiment by stroking from the centre outward or from the eyebrows up to the hair line. Try stroking with both hands or using your hands alternately, stroking one after the other. Find which you like the best. Repeat at least six times.

✱ Massage can help control your pain. It releases chemicals known as endorphins, which are the body's natural pain-killers, and sends them racing around the body to alleviate your suffering.

Eye circling

This movement helps relieve the tension that often builds up around the area leading to eye strain and headaches. Be careful not to drag the skin around this delicate area.

Use the pads of one or two fingers to stroke from the centre of your brow along your eyebrows and around the top of your cheeks to form large, comforting circles around your eyes.

Loosening a tight jaw

If you tend to clench your teeth when under stress, this sequence will be especially beneficial.

1 Place your hands at the sides of your mouth. Stroke the heels of your hands outward to the ears three or four times.

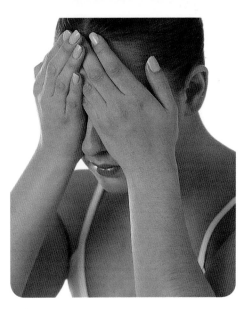

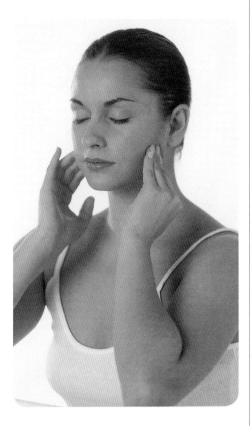

2 Now make small kneading rotations over the same area using the pads of your two middle fingers. Feel for any taut muscles. Move smoothly around the area to warm and soften the powerful jaw muscles that often become stiff and tense. Finish by stroking the area again.

ℐ⬝ *A tight scalp is a sure sign of stress. When the facial muscles become taut with worry or anger, this causes a tightening in the layer of tissue covering the skull, leading to headaches and eye strain. You can feel the tension by trying to move your scalp. Does it move freely or does it seem glued to the bone? Regular scalp massage helps loosen and relax this layer of tissue, so helping to keep you free from tension headaches.*

Repeat final darkness

Complete your headache routine by repeating the first sequence. Stay in darkness for as long as you wish. If you have the opportunity, rest on a bed in a dimly lit or darkened room for half an hour or so after the massage. This enables your body to direct more energy toward relieving your headache.

Top up your fluid levels

Dehydration is a common cause of headaches. Drinking a glass of cool water regularly will restore the fluid you lose during the day and help flush the toxins from your body. Keep a bottle of water beside you and keep sipping it throughout the day.

ℐ⬝ *A cold compress can also help ease the pain of your headache. Fill a bowl with ice-cold water and add three to four drops of lavender oil. Place a folded face flannel on the water and let it absorb the oil floating on the surface. Wring out the flannel so that it is moist but not wet and apply it to the painful area for about fifteen minutes. Renew as necessary. Chilled eye masks are also wonderfully soothing, or place two slices of cold cucumber over your eyes.*

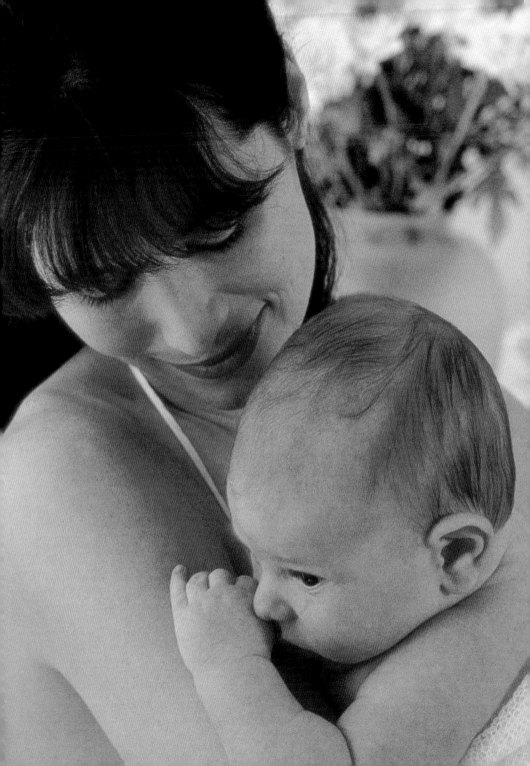

CHAPTER NINE

FAMILY FOCUS

E VERYONE CAN BENEFIT from Indian head massage – from the very young to the very old – not only physically but emotionally too. Enjoying the pleasure of a caring touch brings tremendous comfort and a sense of security that helps establish a warm and loving atmosphere in the home.

❧ The early days

The desire to nurture and be nurtured is innate. Babies and toddlers love to be cuddled, held and stroked and, as parents, we instinctively want to nurture and caress our offspring. Nature certainly knows best. Research in orphanages in Romania confirms that physical affection is crucial to a child's health and well-being. Lack of close physical contact in the first few years can hinder emotional, physiological and social development. By contrast, infants who are held, rocked and cuddled tend to be happier and more contented, throw fewer tantrums, suffer less colic, eat better and sleep more soundly.

The benefits of a loving touch can be extended still further by giving your baby a regular massage and continuing this practice throughout her childhood. Studies now show that massaging premature babies can help stimulate their growth and the development of their immune systems so that they gain more weight and thrive. The positive effects of massage, for both parents and children, are now so widely recognized in the West that most new mothers, and fathers too, are actively encouraged to share the soothing, loving experience.

The following sequence is for a quick and simple face, head, shoulder and arm massage. It is designed to introduce you to the pleasures of baby and infant massage. There is no need to make it a formal session, or to follow the steps rigidly. Aim to discover your child's likes and dislikes. You can massage your baby or toddler whenever you both feel like having some close contact with each other. Before or after bathing is a very popular time because this is such a lovely, cosy moment. She can be fully undressed or wearing a nappy, as you wish. But do make sure that she does not get cold. Stop as soon as your baby becomes fractious or seems to be no longer enjoying herself, and try again another time.

❧ *If you would like to know more about sharing the many benefits of full-body massage with your baby, ask your health visitor to recommend a class in your area. You will be able to massage your baby, with an expert on hand to guide you.*

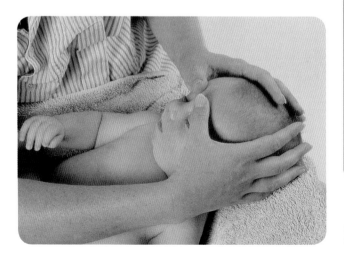

Until the age of about two or three, a baby's skull is very delicate and must be handled extremely carefully. Never press heavily on the skin or hair covering the soft areas on the top and sides of the head. These soft areas, called the fontanelles, are the spaces where the skull bones have not yet knitted. The fontanelles allow the bones of the skull to move during birth. The soft bones mould the skull to the shape of the mother's birth canal so that the head can pass down more freely. As your child grows, the skull bones start to fuse together to form a rigid structure.

Take immense care when massaging a baby's delicate head.

Get comfortable

Try out several different positions to find out which one suits you best. Keep your baby facing you. Some options include:

- Sitting on the edge of a cushion with your legs stretched out in front of you in a V shape – with your baby lying on the floor between your legs.

- Sitting on a cushion, your back supported against a wall or heavy piece of furniture, with your baby lying on your lap. Your knees can be bent or straight.

- If you suffer from back pain, try resting your baby on a table or changing unit that is the right height for you. Never leave your baby unattended on a table or other high position.

Loving hold

Very gently, cradle your baby's head in your hands so that she feels secure and sure of your presence. Lightly rest the palms of your hands above her ears, with your fingertips touching at the top of her head. Keep the touch very, very gentle. Hold for a minute or so and establish eye contact.

CAUTIONS ✍ **Do not exert any pressure on your baby's head.**

Facial strokes

1 Support the side of your baby's head with one hand and very gently, slowly and rhythmically stroke the pads of one or two fingers across her forehead. Start at the centre and work out toward the temples.

2 Continue these feather-like strokes from the sides of her nose to her ears and under her chin. Trace a circular pattern over her face with the pad of your fingers, circling her nose, mouth and chin. Gently rub her ears.

Let your baby explore your face too. Encourage her to touch, feel and pat your face and head. If you wear glasses, take them off first!

Smoothing on the oil

1 Put a few drops of a suitable oil in the palm of one hand (half a teaspoon is plenty). Rub your hands together briskly so that they are warm and well lubricated with oil.

2 Gently stroke from the centre of her head down the sides and back of her head to her neck. Take special care to keep your touch very light, gliding over the surface of her skin and hair.

CAUTIONS ✍ **Take extreme care to avoid pressing on the soft spot, or fontanelle, on the top of your baby's head.**

Stroking the arms

1 Rest your hands lightly at the base of your baby's neck and gently stroke over her shoulders and arms with the palms of your hands.

2 Delicately trace small circular strokes with the pads of your fingers, spiralling up the arm. Cover the whole arm with soft strokes. Finish the massage in the starting position with her head cupped between your hands.

🐾 It is no coincidence that babies in India rarely cry – they are in almost constant close physical contact with their mothers. In many parts of India, babies are not taken outside for the first forty days after birth. Instead, they stay close to their mothers in the warmth and peace of the home.

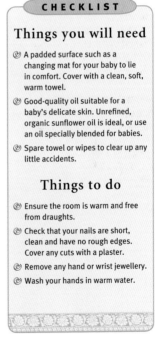

CHECKLIST

Things you will need

- 🖐 A padded surface such as a changing mat for your baby to lie in comfort. Cover with a clean, soft, warm towel.
- 🖐 Good-quality oil suitable for a baby's delicate skin. Unrefined, organic sunflower oil is ideal, or use an oil specially blended for babies.
- 🖐 Spare towel or wipes to clear up any little accidents.

Things to do

- 🖐 Ensure the room is warm and free from draughts.
- 🖐 Check that your nails are short, clean and have no rough edges. Cover any cuts with a plaster.
- 🖐 Remove any hand or wrist jewellery.
- 🖐 Wash your hands in warm water.

☺ Getting your toddler to sleep

Tempers can easily get frayed at bedtime. The following simple, impromptu massage movements may help your toddler get to sleep when she is over-tired and fractious. You do not need any oil, so your child can stay in bed in her pyjamas.

Peace and quiet

Sit on the bed with your back resting against the bed-head or wall. Prop yourself up with pillows, if you will feel more comfortable. Your child sits between your outstretched legs with her head against your chest. You may like to support her back with a small cushion or rolled-up towel.

1 Ask your child to shut her eyes – often not as easy as it sounds. It may help to try sprinkling some imaginary sleepy dust on her eyes to close them but if she refuses to co-operate then she could just look at a book.

2 Rest the palms of your hands gently on her forehead, at the hairline, with your fingers slightly overlapping in the middle. Stay like this for a minute or so. It is very calming and allows you both to enjoy some stillness and peace. Breathe calmly and slowly. Listen as her breathing starts to follow yours.

🍂 *As you massage, smile, talk softly or sing quietly. Try to keep one hand in contact with her skin at all times. Focus on your breathing. Take deep, even breaths. Your child is very receptive to your moods, so try to stay as calm, confident and relaxed as possible.*

Sleepy stroking

1 Place your hands on the top of her head and slowly and gently stroke down either side of her head to her ears. Repeat several times. Repetition is wonderfully reassuring. Sing or hum very softly.

2 Place the palms of your hands on her forehead and make some gentle circles in the centre above the eyebrows. Now stroke from the centre outward. You can use one hand – or two hands, alternating the strokes so that one stroke flows smoothly into the next. Keep the movements very slow and loving. Repeat as many times as you like. Continue these gentle smoothing glides all over her face, working from the centre outward. Imagine that you are stroking her cares away.

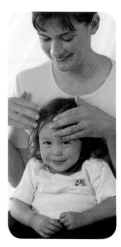

Repeat the first step of "Sleepy stroking" and finish by repeating step two of "Peace and quiet".

🍂 *If your baby or child seems continually upset and crying all the time, when she does not seem unwell and there is no obvious cause of her distress, consider consulting a cranial osteopath (see page 107), who may be able to help.*

✿ Growing up with Indian head massage

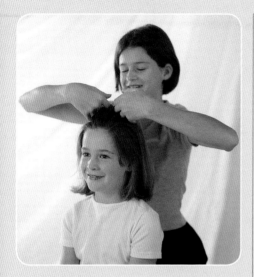

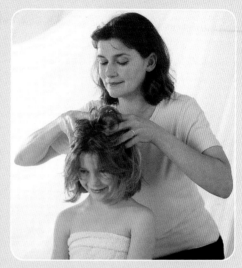

✤ Children are often more sensitive than we think and can get just as stressed as adults, sometimes even more so. Our modern world is full of pressures, choices and expectations. Young people are bombarded with the frenzy and noise of television, computers and video games. They may also have worries about friendships, homework, bullying and disturbing items on the news. Sometimes it can all get too much – leading to mental, physical and emotional overload. Frequent headaches, stomach upsets and muscle twitches are all signs of stress in children.

✤ **Children over the age of about eight are often reluctant to be seen hugging or kissing their parents or siblings in public. However, when you are on your own together, they usually love the comfort of an arm around their shoulders and may well sit on your knee, especially when they are feeling tired or upset. Close physical contact with someone you love is a powerful way of soothing troubles and boosting confidence. The caring, relaxing sensation of an Indian head massage shared within the family may encourage the release of any feelings or concerns that are being bottled up inside.**

✤ The massage movements on the previous pages can be adapted for children over about three years of age.

If they fidget and wriggle, use a lighter pressure and reduce the length of the massage. Most children generally do not like having oil in their hair, so it may be better to give a dry massage or use a very small amount of oil. It is virtually impossible to plan a session, so grab the opportunity when you are both in the mood for massage. This might be first thing in the morning, at bedtime, or any time during the day that your child seems to need some extra love and attention. Do not force your child; judge the right time.

Stormy times

It can be difficult being a teenager. This is a time of intense doubts, fears and inner turmoil. The change from childhood to adulthood can be very daunting, lonely and bewildering – with uncertainties about physical development, hormonal changes, relationship difficulties and the pressure of exams and career choices. A hectic lifestyle, fast-food diet and late nights only make matters worse. Although many parents and adolescents may seem to be at loggerheads most of the time, current studies show that they still usually hold a great affection for each other – they just do not always know how to show it.

Sharing an Indian head massage can be a way of helping you both to relax, unwind and look at your problems and

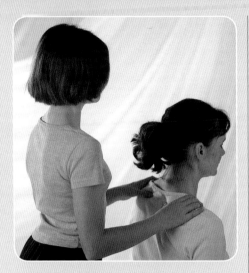

prompt her on occasion, however, so that you can enjoy your favourite moves with the right depth of pressure. Do make it very clear that the spine must always be avoided. All you need to do then is rest and unwind as she kneads your shoulders, "shampoos" your hair and rubs your back.

♣ Next time you are feeling uptight and stressed, ask your child or teenager for a massage – you will both feel a lot calmer and happier afterward.

Bridging the generation gap
In India, grandparents often ask their grandchildren for a massage to relieve their aches and pains. Massage can also be a way of forging a bond between family members of different generations – and a time to exchange news and stories. Many elderly people, especially those living on their own, have little physical contact with others. This can lead to feelings of isolation, depression and loss of self-esteem. A caring touch from a child can make all the difference. Although some children may be hesitant about cuddling their grandparents, they may find the more formal approach of touch through massage quite acceptable – even great fun. Your child can enjoy trying out the different massage techniques that he has already practised on you, although he may need to have a lighter and less vigorous approach if the grandparent is rather frail.

disagreements from another point of view. It can help rekindle a bond between you and provide emotional warmth and security to help you work through this difficult stage. Professional therapists are now being invited into some secondary schools to help boost the pupils' concentration and combat tiredness and exam stress. You can use some of the techniques from the previous pages to do the same in your own home – and ask your teenager to give you a massage, too!

Rubbing parents up the right way
Most children of around seven or eight years of age can give a very firm, relaxing and caring massage. Indeed, children often enjoy giving more than receiving. Think how they instinctively use their tactile senses to explore the world and how they love to rearrange your hair and softly stroke your face. They have few inhibitions about touch and find it perfectly natural to communicate love and affection through their hands. Most children enjoy experimenting with different moves and feel very proud of their achievements when you praise their efforts.

You will need to try out different positions for massaging, depending on your child's height. One of the most comfortable positions is sitting on a cushion on the floor, with your child sitting on a chair or kneeling on a cushion behind you. It is probably best that your child massages without oil, or uses only a tiny amount of oil, as you could both get rather messy. If you have already massaged your child, she may be able to copy your movements without any tuition. You may like to

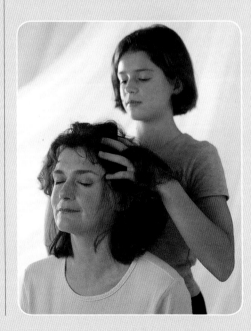

☻ Cranial osteopathy

Many people ask if there is any similarity between Indian head massage and cranial osteopathy. In fact, the two are completely different therapies. Cranial osteopathy was developed in the 1930s by a US osteopath, Dr William Garner Sutherland. It is a highly specialized therapy that works by gentle manipulation of the bones in the cranium, the dome-shaped part of the skull that protects the brain. It is a common misconception that the cranium is one continuous bone. It is not. The cranium is made up of several bones that are connected by interlocking joints.

Therapists claim to be able to sense by touch the rhythm of the cerebrospinal fluid, which nourishes and protects the membranes that encase the brain and spinal cord. This fluid is said to pulsate at between 6–15 times per minute but can be disturbed by pressure on the head and injuries and tensions in the body. This cranial rhythmic impulse (CRI) is difficult to measure, but qualified practitioners have been trained to use delicate manipulation of the cranial and spinal bones to restore it to its correct rhythm. Blood circulation is also boosted and lymph and sinus fluids in the head are drained.

Cranial osteopathy can be used on adults to help problems

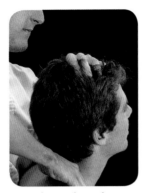

A cranial osteopath at work.

ranging from stress to physical pain. However, it is a particularly useful therapy for young children, when it is often known as paediatric osteopathy. It has been shown to relieve colic, glue ear and recurrent infections. It can even be used on babies to correct cranial bone distortions caused during a difficult birth. Early treatment, when a child's cranial bones are particularly flexible, can prevent problems later in life.

Craniosacral therapy grew out of cranial osteopathy but is more concerned with soft tissue than with bones. Founded in the 1970s by a Michigan State University osteopath, Dr John Upledger, it works on the principle that the CRI affects the whole body through the connective tissues that link all the organs, bones and muscles.

Practitioners believe that it is the membranes encasing the brain and spinal cord that generate the CRI. Using subtle hand pressure on the body, usually around the head or base of the spine, they identify and relieve pain and tension and thereby re-establish an even, rhythmic flow of CRI. Unlike cranial osteopathy, the cranium is not manipulated.

Craniosacral therapy, which is widely practised in the US, can help nervous problems, pain and even paralysis. Patients also report feelings of deep relaxation and the release of tension.

CASE STUDY

Baby blues

Ruth, 30, was so exhausted after the birth of her baby, Joe, that she rarely had the energy to get dressed before midday. "I had expected to be all excited and motherly but I missed my job and social life and spent most of my time in tears," she explained. "I looked a mess – my hair was all over the place and my skin was spotty. Then my mobile hairdresser said that she could give me an Indian head massage, which may help boost my morale and improve the condition of my hair and skin. It was the most wonderful feeling when she stroked my hair and face. I could almost feel the stress lifting. When I looked in the mirror afterward, it was quite different person looking back. Far less strained and more relaxed.

"My hairdresser came back several times to give me a weekly head massage and always made time for a chat afterward. Her caring touch and interest in my well-being helped me rebuild my confidence and I began to enjoy motherhood. She told me how to massage my own head using oils to help my hair regain strength after pregnancy and has really made a difference.

"She also suggested that I should try to massage baby Joe. Massage is now part of our bath-time ritual – he gurgles and smiles at me and we have a lot of fun. I still have my ups and downs but as soon as I start to feel low again I book in for a head massage to raise my spirits and put some colour in my cheeks."

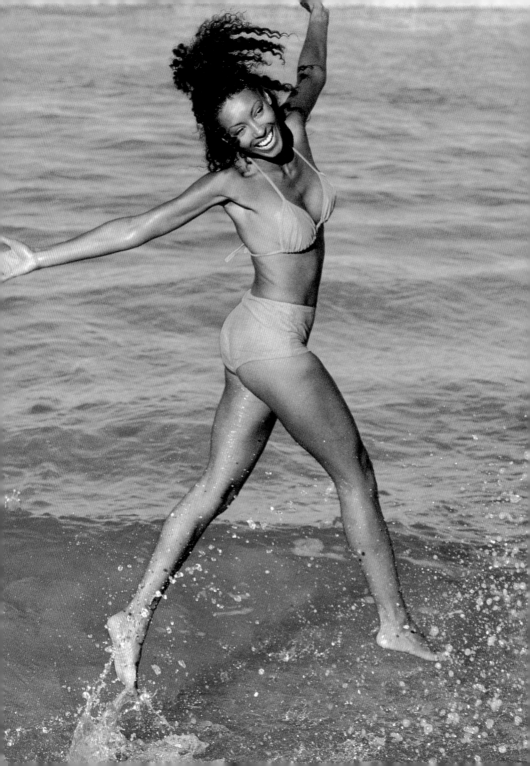

CHAPTER TEN

A HEALTHY LIFESTYLE

R EGULAR INDIAN HEAD MASSAGE can often inspire a greater sense of self-awareness and enthusiasm for a healthier, less stressful lifestyle. As your friends and family start to appreciate the interaction of mind and body they may also show a positive interest in taking responsibility for their own health and well-being. It is useful to be able to offer some general tips and suggestions for a healthier way of life. Do not forget to follow your own advice!

☙ Reactions to Indian head massage

Your massage partner may experience a range of mild reactions, known as contra-actions, during or immediately after an Indian head massage. These are different for each person and may vary on each occasion. Any transient reactions should be regarded as a positive indication that the body is rebalancing and cleansing itself – they are often a consequence of the body clearing out toxins that may have built up over a long period of time.

Common reactions during treatment

These contra-actions can be rather off-putting at first, so be aware of the most common ones and offer reassurance in advance. Once any initial mild ill-effects have passed, your massage partner should feel in much better health.

☙ Tell your massage partner not to fight sleep. His body needs it. Ensure that you are giving his head maximum support and continue the massage as usual. Gently awaken him at the end of the massage and allow time for him to "come round". He may feel quite disorientated for a while.

☙ It is not unusual for people to become quite tearful, angry or giggly during or after an Indian head massage. This is not a cause for embarrassment – laughing, shedding tears and shouting are wonderfully effective tension-busters and should be encouraged if your partner is feeling tense. Be open to sharing any problems, without being seen to interfere or judge. Be sensitive to the mood and ask if your massage partner would like you to continue or stop and talk. It may prove a perfect opportunity to discuss any concerns.

☙ Some people can suddenly feel hot and flushed or tingly as blood circulation is increased to the head and upper back. Others may feel cold and shivery as body temperature falls with general relaxation. Look out for body language and tune in to your massage partner's needs. Turn down the heat in the room or provide another towel for extra warmth. If your partner feels light-headed or dizzy, offer a glass of water and suggest that he rests a while before getting up from the chair.

❧ *Contra-actions are normal and should not last for more than two to three days. Encourage your partner to resist the temptation to suppress any aches, pains or other natural reactions*

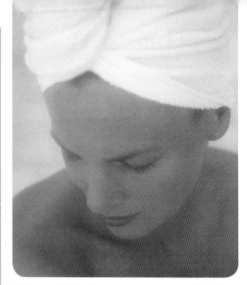

If oils are used during the massage wrap your partner's head in a warm towel for a while before washing.

to Indian head massage with over-the-counter medicines. Often conditions can get a little worse before they get better.

Common reactions after treatment

☙ Some people suffer varying degrees of tiredness. This is a signal that mind and body need rest to recuperate and recharge. Tell your partner not to ignore the signs. Suggest that he goes to bed for a few hours, if possible, rather than forcing himself to keep up a hectic pace of life. This post-massage tiredness usually lifts after the first few massages. Try to make the next massage in the early evening when there is more chance of resting afterward. Others feel a remarkable surge of energy after an Indian head massage – but do warn your partner not to over-do things or there is a risk of getting overtired.

☙ This contra-action passes, too, after a few massages. It is usually due to the release of toxins into the bloodstream or it may be a response to deep work on the muscle fibres. Occasionally, people may suffer some transient nausea or dizziness. Encourage your partner to drink plenty of water to help flush the toxins through the body.

☙ This can take several forms including more frequent bowel movements and urination (there may be some change in colour or odour). Your partner may also notice slightly increased perspiration, possibly a mild skin rash and an excess of mucus.

☙ After massage

☙ If you used oils when you gave the massage, wrap your partner's head in a warm towel for at least half an hour before washing.

☙ Ask your massage partner to be still for a few minutes to enjoy the benefits of the massage. Suggest she takes it easy for the next twelve hours to ensure energy is directed toward helping the body to heal itself. She should rest as much as possible and avoid strenuous exercise.

☙ Advise her to drink plenty of still tap or mineral water and herbal teas to speed up the elimination of toxins from the body. She should also cut back on tea, coffee and colas, which act like a diuretic (increasing the flow of urine out of the body), and try not to smoke or drink alcohol for at least twelve hours to allow the body to detoxify itself.

☙ Heavy meals should also be avoided straight after a massage. The demands of digestion will divert energy away from the natural healing process. Light snacks, fresh fruit or raw vegetables are ideal.

☙ Your partner should take particular care when driving – deep relaxation may cause her reactions to be temporarily slower. If she feels light-headed, ask her to wait until she feels ready to drive and suggest that she keeps the window open.

☙ Control your breathing

Breathing comes so naturally that most people do not give it a second thought. However, poor breathing can contribute to many health conditions ranging from dizzy spells and general lethargy to heart problems. Calm controlled breathing, on the other hand, increases your intake of oxygen, providing the energy you need for the proper functioning of every cell in the body, including the brain. The circulation of fully reoxygenated blood around the body boosts energy levels, relieves stress and helps you to think with greater clarity.

Bad breathing habits are often caused by a number of factors including poor posture, lack of exercise and a build-up of stress – which can all be corrected with a healthy lifestyle. Restrictive clothing can also hinder breathing, so avoid tight belts and waistlines. The most common fault is fast, shallow breathing, which means that the lungs are not being used to their full capacity. If breathing is not deep enough, inhaled air is not drawn down to the lower lungs where most of the blood circulates. Not only do you miss out on your full quota of fresh oxygen, but carbon dioxide and other waste products are not being totally removed.

When you are breathing effectively, the movement comes from the diaphragm, not the chest. The diaphragm, the dome-like muscle that divides the chest and abdomen, pushes downward to allow more air to flow deep down into the lungs.

☙ Exercise for energy

Our lifestyles have generally become increasingly sedentary over recent years. We tend to travel by car or bus, use labour-saving equipment and spend hours in front of the television or computer. So it is important to include regular physical activity in the daily routine. Regular exercise improves blood circulation, strengthens and tones muscles, encourages deep breathing, boosts the immune system and helps prevent a number of serious medical conditions including heart disease and osteoporosis. Exercise also releases tension and

Regular exercise will help improve your physical well-being in so many ways.

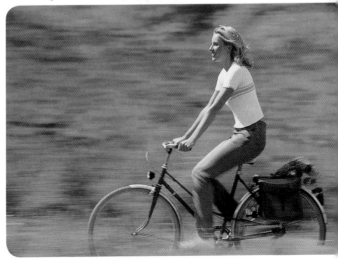

Are you breathing correctly?

⊛ Lie flat on the floor. Place one hand on your chest and the other on your abdomen. Your chest should be almost still and the hand on your abdomen should rise and fall in a rhythmic fashion. With slow, deep breathing the rate of breaths per minute usually falls from fifteen to about twelve.

Giving up smoking is possibly the single most important step you can take to improve your general health and prevent future illness. It is much easier said than done – but enjoying the benefits of regular Indian head massage may provide the perfect motivation to kick the habit – or at least to cut down. Keep reminding yourself of the benefits of giving up. Picture yourself feeling more energetic, positive and happy with glowing skin and shiny hair.

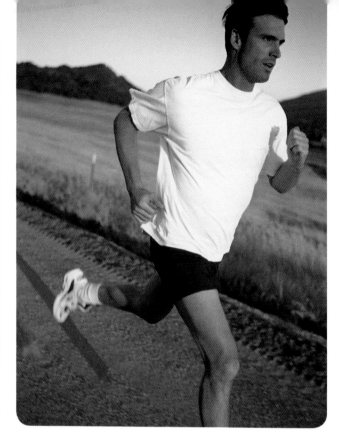

Keep yourself healthy by exercising on a regular basis.

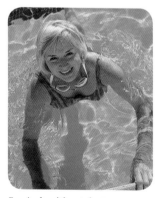

Exercise doesn't have to be strenuous – a gentler activity is just as beneficial.

combats fatigue. Many people who exercise regularly find that they are far more alert and energetic after exercise than before.

Be moderate

You do not need to sweat it out in the gym or on the squash court to reap the rewards of regular exercise. Around thirty minutes of moderate exercise carried out three to five times a week is the recommended prescription for good health. This can be any form of activity that you enjoy – swimming, brisk walking, dancing, housework and gardening are all ideal – so long as it raises your heartbeat and leaves you warm and slightly out of breath.

The suggested half an hour of activity can be taken in one session or accumulated during the day. Even small moves toward a more active lifestyle can bring significant health benefits: think twice about taking the car on short journeys, boycott the escalator, run up the stairs and put some extra elbow-grease into cleaning the windows.

Mind and body exercise

Many people enjoy significant benefits from taking part in an activity that exercises both mind and body – such as tai chi or hatha yoga. Regular practice will aid good posture, controlled breathing, self-awareness and relaxation to bring harmony and balance to your life. These activities also promote flexibility, increase strength and help maintain and restore good health and well-being. Some inverted yoga postures even complement Indian head massage by stimulating blood flow to the scalp.

Are you fit enough?

Walk up and down a flight of stairs three times – about fifteen steps is sufficient. At the end you should have enough breath to carry on a conversation. Stop if you feel dizzy, sick or uncomfortable during the test. While exercising, use the talk test to check you are working at the right level. You should still be able to chat. If you are gasping for breath then you are over-exerting yourself; if you can sing you are taking it too easy.

☺ Get enough sleep

Everyone needs different amounts of sleep. The average is around seven to eight hours a night but we tend to need less as we get older. However, it is not necessarily the number of hours but the quality of your sleep that matters most. If you are getting too much sleep, you will feel sluggish. If you are getting too little, you will feel drained, tense and tetchy. A restful night's sleep repairs and restores the tissues of the body, rests and relaxes the mind and strengthens the immune system. You wake up feeling refreshed and ready to tackle the challenges of the day ahead. When you do not get enough sleep, however, you tend to feel irritable, lethargic and muzzy-headed. Your skin and hair become dry and lifeless and you may start to feel depressed and anxious.

A good night's sleep can work wonders in improving your general well-being.

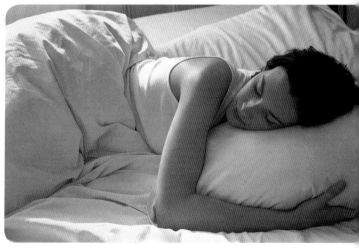

Beating sleeplessness

If you are finding that sleeplessness or disturbed sleep is becoming a problem, there are some simple measures that you can try. Set up a sleep routine with a regular bedtime and waking hour and avoid taking naps during the day. Establish some pre-sleep "winding-down" routines, such as relaxing in a warm bath, reading a book or magazine that is not too mentally stimulating – or have a soothing Indian head massage. Avoid vigorous exercise just before retiring to bed (sex is an exception as this can act as a natural and pleasurable sedative!). Make your bedroom a calm, relaxing sanctuary. Get rid of all the distracting clutter and keep it well-ventilated and at a comfortable temperature. If you wake up feeling cold, put on some socks and an extra top. Wear ear plugs if it is too noisy, or an eye mask if it is too light.

Banish worry

Try to rest quietly and think of pleasant thoughts such as planning a holiday or painting a picture. Monotonous mind games, like counting backward from 200, can sometimes help divert your thoughts. Listen to your breathing or practise a favourite relaxation technique (see page 60) to stop your mind buzzing. Try not to worry about the lack of sleep. The occasional sleepless night is perfectly normal. It only becomes harmful when you go for weeks or months without sleep. If you still cannot get to sleep, try not to toss and turn and fret. Get out of bed for around fifteen minutes and do something constructive – perhaps iron some clothes, jot down some notes or make yourself a drink of warm milk.

CHECKLIST

Healthy food habits

- ☺ Choose natural, fresh food. Avoid food packed with preservatives, flavourings and colourings.
- ☺ Buy lean cuts of meat. Trim off the fat before eating.
- ☺ Eat regularly to maintain blood sugar levels. Never skip meals.
- ☺ Study food labels so you can make healthy choices.
- ☺ Steam vegetables – rather than frying or boiling them – to retain nutrients.
- ☺ Most importantly, take time to sit down and really enjoy your food.

☺ Eat and drink for health

There is no doubt that a sensible diet, full of essential nutrients, is vital for maintaining good health and preventing ill health. Following a well-balanced diet need not be complicated or obsessive; it is a question of following a few simple guidelines that form the basis of good nutrition.

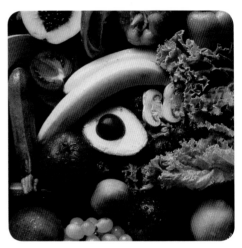

Eat as much fresh produce as possible to maintain a healthy diet.

Vary your food intake so you have a mixed diet. Eat at least five portions of fresh fruit and vegetables every day preferably organic. For the best effects, eat them raw as that way the vitamins and minerals are retained. Balance your diet so that around half your intake comprises starchy complex carbohydrates such as pasta, bread, oats, potatoes and rice. Avoid severe calorie-restricted diets as you could be missing out on essential nutrients, which leaves you feeling tired and irritable with poor memory and concentration.

Cut down on fat

Limit your fat intake to less than a third of your daily number of calories. Cut right back on foods rich in saturated fat – mainly in red meat, processed foods and full-fat dairy products, such as cheese, whole milk and cream. Aim to eat more foods high in unsaturated fats – fish, especially salmon, mackerel and sardines, nuts and seeds. Dress salads in unrefined cold-pressed oils such as sunflower, olive, grapeseed, sesame, walnut and corn.

Have less sugar – and watch out for hidden sugar in convenience and processed foods. If you need an energy-boost, choose a banana, sandwich, cracker or bowl of cereal. Eat more fibre. Choose wholemeal bread, cereals, rice and pasta and eat plenty of pulses. Keep your alcohol intake within sensible limits. Aim to have at least three alcohol-free days a week.

Water works

Increasing your intake of water can make a major difference to your health and appearance. Even mild dehydration can cause tiredness, headaches, dry skin, constipation and lapses of concentration. Around 75 per cent of the body is made up of water. It is necessary for every bodily function, including breathing and thinking. Water carries vital nutrients around the body to all the living cells and flushes out toxic residues. We lose around three litres of water a day through perspiration, respiration and urination. Some of this is replaced by fluid in the food we eat, but not all. So it is necessary to drink enough water to top up the fluid levels and keep the body running smoothly.

Avoid dehydration by drinking lots of water.

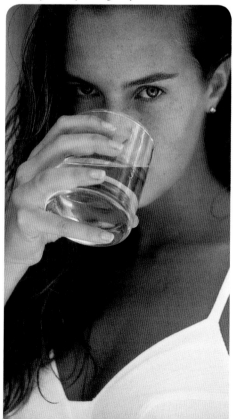

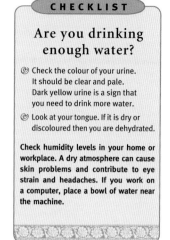

CHECKLIST

Are you drinking enough water?

- Check the colour of your urine. It should be clear and pale. Dark yellow urine is a sign that you need to drink more water.
- Look at your tongue. If it is dry or discoloured then you are dehydrated.

Check humidity levels in your home or workplace. A dry atmosphere can cause skin problems and contribute to eye strain and headaches. If you work on a computer, place a bowl of water near the machine.

The recommended daily dose of water is around 1.8 litres (eight glasses), although you may need to drink a little more at times of stress or anxiety when there are high demands on your body. Keep a bottle of water at home, at work and in the car so that you can take sips through the day. Do not wait until your mouth feels dry – drink at regular intervals. Ordinary tea, coffee and colas do not count as part of your fluid quota. Quite the reverse, in fact, as they do not stay in the body long enough to do the job. They act as diuretics that stimulate the kidneys to excrete even more water in your urine. You should aim to drink one extra cup of water to compensate for every cup of coffee or tea.

Try drinking herbal teas to add variety to your fluid intake. Peppermint and chamomile teas are very relaxing. Nettle and dandelion teas are said to help healthy hair growth. Ginger tea is highly regarded within the Ayurvedic system as it is reputed to stimulate blood circulation and aid digestion.

Are you the right weight?

If you are already following most of the above suggestions, you are probably in pretty good shape. However, you may also like to check that you are maintaining a healthy weight for your height by working out your body mass index (BMI). Divide your weight in kilograms by your height in metres squared. Your BMI should be between 20 and 25. If it is over 30, your weight could seriously affect your health. This calculation is not suitable for children or teenagers.

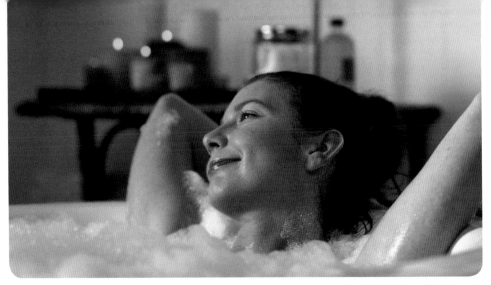

A soothing bath is one of the best ways to relax and relieve stress.

⊛ Learn to handle stress

Stress is an inevitable part of life (see page 29). You cannot avoid it, but you can learn how to manage difficult situations in a calm and composed state of mind.

Try to identify and recognize the circumstances and people that make you feel frustrated, irritated and pressurized and work out strategies for avoiding them or limiting their negative effect on you.

Take five

Take a break during your lunch hour – anything to interrupt the routine and change the scene. If you feel that you are becoming stressed, try to go somewhere peaceful. Count to ten, have a good stretch, listen to some calming music or practise a relaxation exercise (see page 60). After work, take a few minutes alone to wind down so worries do not spoil your evening. Do not miss out on your annual holiday entitlement.

Manage your time

Stress is often caused by things that you know you ought to do, so do not put them off – tackle them now. Try to deal with paperwork and bills as soon as they arrive. However, be realistic about your targets. Plan your jobs and put them in order of priority. Try to allow plenty of time so that you do not need to rush. Learn to say "no" to demands and delegate as much as possible.

Pamper yourself

Follow the guidelines over the previous pages. A good night's sleep, regular exercise and a well-balanced diet can help keep stress levels under control. Set time aside for yourself, away from responsibilities, to do something totally for yourself. Pamper yourself – book in for a facial, read a book, luxuriate in a warm bath or phone a friend for a long chat. A weekly Indian head massage is ideal.

> ### CHECKLIST
>
> ## Are you stressed?
>
> When you are finding it hard to cope with the stresses in your life, you may notice the following changes in your emotions and behaviour.
>
> - ⊛ Feelings of guilt when relaxing.
> - ⊛ Difficulty in getting to sleep or waking early.
> - ⊛ Impatience, irritability, intolerance of others, frequent arguments.
> - ⊛ Low self-esteem.
> - ⊛ Lack of appetite or over-eating.
> - ⊛ Excessive smoking and drinking.
> - ⊛ Nail-biting and teeth-grinding.
> - ⊛ Difficulty in concentrating and making decisions.
> - ⊛ Tension in the muscles of your neck, upper back and shoulders.
> - ⊛ Loss of interest in sex.
> - ⊛ Frequent headaches.

Simple enjoyment

Enjoy the simple pleasures in life – a child's smile, a butterfly floating through the sky or the sun rising at dawn. Smile and be pleasant to others. Surround yourself with friends or family whom you love and trust. Share any worries or troubles with those people you can rely on for positive support.

Have fun

A good laugh is brilliant therapy. A bout of laughing has been shown to relax tense muscles, soothe stress, deepen breathing, improve blood circulation, boost the immune system and encourage the release of "happiness" hormones. It has even been referred to as "internal aerobics" because it speeds up the metabolic rate and provides excellent exercise. Search out friends and situations that make you laugh. Re-read a funny article in a magazine or watch a favourite comedy video. Try making yourself laugh out loud by remembering something amusing that happened to you.

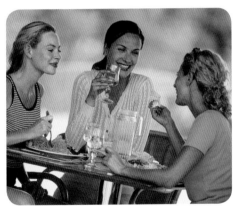

Make time to enjoy the sunshine and have a laugh with friends.

Enjoy some sunlight

The winter blues are often caused by lack of sunlight. A more serious problem, known as seasonal affective disorder (SAD); with symptoms including lethargy, anxiety and loss of self-esteem, is directly linked with the gloomy days of autumn and winter. Boost energy levels, lower stress levels and balance your levels of vitamin D by enjoying at least thirty minutes of natural daylight every day. It is surprising how much more alert and alive you feel afterward. But do wear adequate protection against the harmful rays of the sun.

✆ Hair care tips

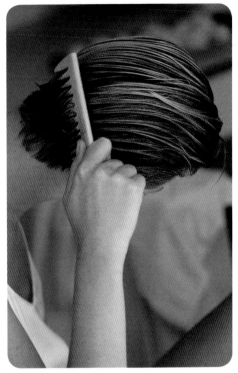

Use a wide-toothed comb on wet hair.

Some gentle care and attention with regular scalp massage using moisturizing vegetable carrier oils helps keep hair strong, shiny and easy to manage. Wash your hair frequently (two or three times a week) to keep the hair and scalp clean and free from debris. Wet your hair thoroughly. Use a small amount of gentle shampoo that has been formulated to suit your hair type. Rinse well afterward to ensure that your hair is free from any residue of lather. Use a suitable mild conditioner and rinse in clear, warm water.

Take care

Wet hair can easily be broken. Use a wide-toothed comb. Start with the ends and then work up to the roots. Limit blow drying as this can dry out and damage your hair. Allow your hair to dry naturally, away from direct sunlight, after wrapping it in a towel and squeezing out the excess water. If you are using a dryer, set it to medium heat and hold it a little distance away from your head.

How good is your posture?

Take a good look at yourself in a full-length mirror. Your weight should be evenly distributed, with your feet flat on the ground, knees pointing straight ahead. Your shoulders should be relaxed and at the same height. From the side there should be a straight line that runs from the top of your head, through your ears, arms, hip joints and knees to your feet. There should be a gentle curve in your lower back with your chin neither tucked in nor protruding forward.

POSTURE TIPS

Working at a computer

- Have your chair – and desk, if possible – set to the correct height, your wrists level with or lower than your elbows.
- Sit with your feet flat on the ground, legs uncrossed.
- Sit square to the computer screen so you do not have to twist. Tilt the screen up a little to avoid squinting.
- Take regular breaks – get up and walk around for a few minutes every hour or so. Move your neck slowly from side to side or in gentle forward semi-circles to release tension.
- To avoid eye strain, try not to stare at the screen continuously. Allow your eye muscles to relax by focusing on distant objects.

Driving a car

- Check the height of the seat. You should be able to see clearly over the steering wheel without straining.
- Position the seat so you are not cramped and can reach the controls with ease.
- Sit with the base of your back fully against the seat back. Sit on your buttocks, not your spine.
- Hold the steering wheel fairly loosely, with your hands resting a little lower than your shoulders. Do not grip the wheel tightly, with your hands near the top of the wheel.

Brush regularly, using a brush with natural bristles, to distribute the natural oils and stimulate blood circulation to the scalp. Do not be too rough or you could cause breakage and damage, stress the roots and aggravate scalp conditions. Clean brushes and combs weekly to avoid spreading dirt and grime through the hair.

Protect your hair

Avoid using strong hair sprays and setting agents, which can dry out your hair and make it coarse, brittle and dull. Wear a sun hat or swimming hat or use a protective hair agent to protect your hair from the sun and when swimming in the sea or a chlorinated pool. Rinse your hair thoroughly in fresh water after swimming. Both salt and chlorine are dehydrating if left to dry on the hair. Avoid using curling tongs, heated rollers or chemical processes such as perming, crimping or tinting that can damage and dehydrate your hair. Get your hair trimmed regularly to reduce tangles and split ends. Above all, aim for a well-balanced diet, regular exercise and good-quality sleep.

Check your posture

Poor posture while sitting hunched over a computer or driving a car are common causes of shoulder and neck tension, leading to stiffness, poor circulation, headaches, eye strain and shallow breathing. Good posture can change the way you look and feel, giving you confidence and helping you move with comfort and grace. Correcting your posture does not mean adopting a rigid military pose, which can be just as harmful as slouching. Instead, you should lengthen and widen your spine, keeping your shoulders relaxed.

Think of lifting your breastbone to open up your rib cage. Picture your head balanced evenly and freely on top of your spine, with your limbs extending from the centre, allowing ease of movement. Try to be aware of any tensions in your muscles and learn to relax them and realign your body. If you are interested in improving your posture, consider taking lessons in the Alexander technique (see page 119).

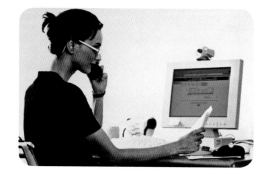

✍ Alexander technique

The Alexander technique was developed by the Australian actor Frederick Alexander in the early 1830s. It is the perfect complement to Indian head massage and helps correct any misalignment between the head, neck and spine. Such misalignments often lead to a wide variety of problems ranging from headaches, migraine and chronic back pain to postural pain in pregnancy and even anxiety and depression.

Birth of a therapy

Alexander found that his voice often became strained and sometimes disappeared altogether during performances and so he began to look for the underlying cause. Studying himself in front of a mirror, he discovered the root of the problem – bad posture. Having taught himself to overcome such bad habits as arching his back before speaking, tensing his arms and legs and tightening his throat muscles, he went on to formalize the technique that bears his name and which has now earned world-wide respect.

Re-learning good posture

We are all affected by years of sitting and standing badly, lifting and bending incorrectly and even walking tensely. Even turning a tap on and off can cause damaging twisting of the back. Small children have beautiful posture, moving with no apparent effort. However, with age we lose this natural posture. Shoulders stoop, spinal misalignment worsens, joints become distorted and bad habits become entrenched. There is also damage caused by repetitive movements, especially at work, and accidents. We can usually learn to live with minor twinges but for some people the pain of musculoskeletal problems can be severe and debilitating.

The Alexander technique teaches you how to identify postural problems and rectify them by allowing the body to re-learn its natural posture. It is not a treatment session, but a course of lessons. The interaction is between teacher and pupil. This is not a massage therapy, and "enjoyment" is not the aim. Nor is relaxation for relaxation's sake, although it may be an end result. It requires a good deal of input from pupils, who are expected to practise the techniques in their daily lives.

Therapy lessons

With practice, there is a release of inappropriate muscle tension and a natural realignment of head, neck and spine.

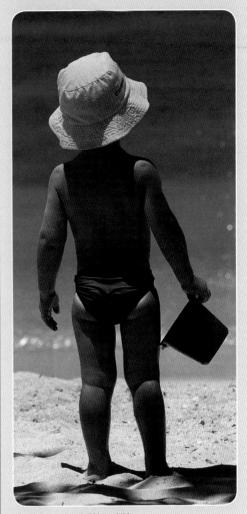

The perfect posture held by a child.

The result is a better balanced and more efficiently functioning body. Pain, even gastrointestinal disorders and breathing problems, can be alleviated. Lessons last 30–45 minutes and a course can consist of 15 to 30 lessons, depending on how quickly the pupil learns and adopts the techniques. Most doctors these days consider the Alexander technique to be helpful, and even some private medical insurance policies cover this therapy.

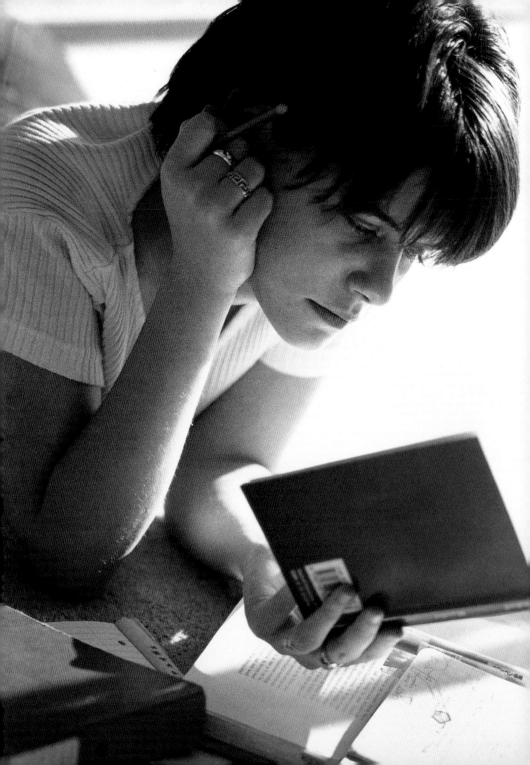

CHAPTER ELEVEN

TAKING IT A STEP FURTHER

I F YOU HAVE ENJOYED practising Indian head massage on family and friends, you may be thinking about developing your massage techniques and knowledge or training to become a professional therapist. There are many short courses and workshops on the subject, run by colleges of further education or by private centres and tutors. Some are also run on a correspondence basis. Courses are structured either for those who simply wish to find out more about this fascinating therapy as a hobby, or those who would like to take Indian head massage more seriously. For many people, Indian head massage can be an extension of their existing qualifications in complementary health, hairdressing or beauty, and may even be a stepping stone to a new career.

To find out more information about courses in your area, look in your local newspaper, search the Internet, telephone nearby colleges that have a health and beauty department or ask at your health food store or natural health centre.

✍ Joining a massage course

A course on Indian head massage provides a great opportunity to meet other people who share a common interest in the health and well-being of others. Learning in a group situation, with the guidance and support of an expert tutor, can be an enlightening, inspiring and refreshing experience. You will find that everyone has something different to offer fellow students – new insights, varied backgrounds and a whole range of talents. It is usually good fun as well as being highly informative, and there is the added bonus that students practise on each other so you will benefit from a regular Indian head massage yourself.

Choosing a course

It is important to select the right level of course for your experience and aspirations. Most colleges and private centres offer preliminary interviews that provide an opportunity to meet your tutor and ask questions – perhaps about the course curriculum, assessment procedure, facilities or pre-entry requirements. Most courses include practical work, often working on a range of clientele. You should also be taught human anatomy and physiology and the safe use of oils. Depending on the length and type of course, you may be expected to carry out case studies at home, complete homework and sit practical, oral and written tests or examinations.

Do not make any commitment or part with any money until you are happy with all the various elements of the course and feel able to establish a good rapport with your particular tutor. It is often a good idea to look at several centres, study different prospectuses and ask for feedback from past and present students before making your final choice. Do be sure that you have the time and energy to attend all the sessions and tackle the tasks within the course. It may be helpful to persuade a friend or your partner to join you. You will then be able to exchange massages, discuss the projects and boost each other's confidence.

Looking the part is important if you are going to be taken seriously.

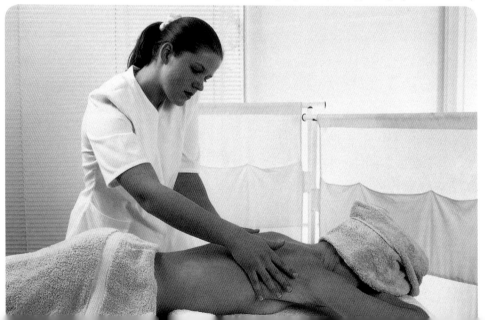

☙ A professional approach

If you would like to set up in business, make sure the training and qualification you will receive are recognized within your industry. Once you have received a practitioner-level qualification, you will then be able to register with an appropriate professional body and obtain insurance. Associations lay down certain obligations including a strict code of ethics or practice and disciplinary procedures that act to reassure the public that you offer a high quality of service. Members of the public are always recommended to check that a practitioner carries the relevant professional qualification, which can be verified by their particular society or organization.

Ask your bank or local enterprise agency for guidance.

Setting up in business

Many people choose to use their qualification in Indian head massage to set up their own small business. If this idea appeals to you, choose a course that has a business element and provides you with the necessary preliminary information to help ensure the success of the venture. You may be expected to draw up a business plan, which will consider issues such as: whether you will work at home, set up a salon or become a mobile therapist; how you will promote and advertise your business; designing brochures and setting charges; purchasing equipment; obtaining the necessary finance to meet initial and on-going expenses – and whether it is a viable financial proposition. If your course does not offer advice, ask your bank or a local enterprise agency for guidance in starting and running a small business.

Career opportunities

Indian head massage is becoming increasingly popular in the West as a health and beauty treatment, with a wide range of options for trained therapists. It is an ideal stress-relieving treatment to offer anyone who has little time to spare or feels inhibited by taking off their clothes for a full-body massage. Hairdressers learn the techniques so they can include a scalp massage in their regular services. Beauticians are now able to offer Indian head massage using a range of oils.

☙ *Completing a course is just the beginning. One of the joys of taking an interest in a subject as varied as complementary medicine is that the learning process never ends. Keep reading books and magazines, practising your techniques, talking to others and attending courses, workshops and exhibitions to stay up-to-date with current ideas, techniques and products.*

Combining therapies

Some complementary health practitioners combine Indian head massage with another therapy such as full body massage, aromatherapy or Reiki, or use some of the movements to relax clients before a treatment such as reflexology. Therapists working in clinics, hospices and rehabilitation centres have found it an extremely beneficial part of a long-term treatment plan. Indian head massage has also been adapted so oils need not be used and clients do not disrobe. Many therapists make regular visits to offices and schools where they give shorter sessions to help relieve tension before an important meeting or exam, or simply to help people cope with the demands of hectic schedules. Indian head massage is also offered as a refreshing pick-me-up on long-haul flights and in VIP lounges at airports.

⊛ Finding a practitioner

If you would like to have a regular Indian head massage, it is a good idea to spend some time finding the right therapist for you. Look at adverts placed in local newspapers and on the Internet – or ask for recommendations from friends, family and work colleagues. Colleges sometimes give special discounts for treatments offered by students as part of their course work – and many clients continue to receive regular massage from these students after they qualify.

When booking an appointment with a therapist it is obviously important to check their level of competence – ask about their training and professional qualifications. Above all, it is essential to find someone whom you trust and respect. You need to feel comfortable and secure with them. A good practitioner will always spend time finding out about your medical history, current health and lifestyle. These details are used to check for contra-indications and work out a treatment plan for your approval. Avoid anyone who offers miracle cures or suggests changing your conventional medicine without consultation with your doctor. Your therapist should have a professional attitude and appearance and answer your questions thoroughly and accurately, giving information about the possible effects.

If you do not feel comfortable with the therapist, try someone else. Trust your judgement. Every practitioner has his or her own personal approach, which may suit some people but not others. Always offer feedback after a treatment so that you are getting exactly the kind of massage you desire – some like it firm and vigorous, others prefer a more gentle, soothing sensation. The choice is yours.

CASE STUDY

Changing careers

When Jackie, 52, a primary school teacher, enrolled on a one-day workshop in Indian head massage, she had no idea that two years later she would be a mobile therapist. "The title of the course captured my imagination," she said. "I wasn't sure what to expect but it sounded interesting – and it was something different to do on a Saturday. However, by the end of the morning session I was so inspired that I didn't want the day to end. I've always loved receiving massage but I never realized that giving massage could be so fulfilling. It was like a whole new world was opening up for me – I felt on a real high and couldn't stop talking about it.

"Since that first workshop, I have done a series of weekend courses to gain my professional qualification in Indian head massage. I have also trained in full-body massage and reflexology and plan to study aromatherapy next year. There is no stopping me. The children have all left home now – so it is the perfect time to change career. At the moment, I'm building up my client base so I can combine teaching with evening and weekend appointments but I eventually hope to give up teaching altogether and set up my own salon at home. Being a complementary therapist may not be as financially rewarding as some occupations, but there is certainly a lot of job satisfaction."

☙ Acupressure, Tui na, Shiatsu

Many Indian head massage therapists incorporate other therapies into their treatments, such as acupressure. This therapy also works on the head, neck and shoulders – as well as other parts of the body – to relieve tension and create harmony of mind and body. Other therapies, such as Tui na and Shiatsu, are also based on acupressure. Each therapy takes a very different approach, however.

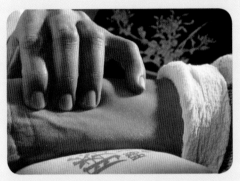

Acupressure is acupuncture without the needles.

Acupressure

This is acupuncture without the needles. Like all traditional forms of Chinese medicine, it can trace its origins back to before 2000 BC and is based on the theory of "qi", or life energy. The practitioner aims to stimulate the flow of qi throughout the body, so relieving ills and promoting health and harmony. Working on channels in the body known as "meridians", the therapist, who is very often an acupuncturist as well, uses fingers and thumbs, and sometimes even feet and knees, to stimulate acupoints and boost qi.

Pressure is often applied in the direction that the meridian flows and acupoints on both sides of the body are massaged to maintain balance. You may feel a slight discomfort when an acupoint is pressed, but overall the therapy is excellent for relieving stress and can help with problems ranging from arthritis to insomnia and from fatigue to digestive disorders. It can also be enjoyed simply as a general health enhancer. With guidance from a therapist, or even a good book, you can practise on yourself.

Tui na

This is the name of the most common form of traditional acupressure practised in China and is gradually becoming known in the West. The name "Tui na" literally means "pushing and grabbing" and refers to the style of clinical massage practised by doctors in hospitals in China. Like acupressure, the guiding principle behind Tui na is that all pain, whether chronic or acute, is the result of an imbalance of qi life energy.

Exponents of Tui na use squeezing, kneading and stroking movements to focus deep pressure along the qi meridians. This is intended to re-energize, invigorate and release blocked energy and allow qi to flow unhindered. The result is relaxed muscles and pain relief. One of its main uses is to treat pain caused by problems of the musculo-skeletal system, such as a slipped disc. In the West, it is now being seen as a useful alternative to orthodox treatments such as anti-inflammatory drugs, prolonged bed rest and even surgery.

Shiatsu

This is also related to acupressure, although far more robust. Its roots are in traditional Chinese medicine and a belief in qi energy, but it was developed in Japan in the early twentieth century and has been greatly influenced by Western medicine. The name "Shiatsu" literally means "finger pressure" and was devised by a Japanese practitioner, Tamai Tempaku, who combined traditional Eastern techniques with an understanding of Western knowledge of physiology and anatomy.

The practice is holistic – seeking to treat the entire body – with treatment usually beginning just below the navel, where it is believed that qi is stored. Practitioners use a wide range of techniques and the session can be extremely physical. Knees, elbows and even feet may be used to stimulate blood and qi flow, employing stretching and squeezing actions to disperse blocked qi and rocking movements to counteract agitated qi. Shiatsu can help with disorders ranging from headaches and migraines to asthma, stress and musculoskeletal pain. It can also be a good general tonic.

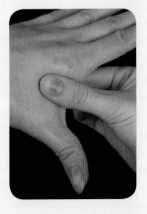

Shiatsu or finger pressure.

Index

Acknowledgements

My interest and enthusiasm for Indian head massage was inspired by my tutors at Chichester College of Arts, Science and Technology – Jo Hammond and Susie Jennings – who have offered invaluable help and advice on this book. I would also like to thank my agent, Chelsey Fox, for her constant encouragement, and my family, friends and clients for sharing their comments and expertise, especially Wendy Bloor, Nina Guilfoyle, Fiona Read, Sarah Salway and Pamela Townsend. My appreciation also to Anita Snowball from the Evadell Natural Therapy Centre, Jennifer Aitken and Bernadette Cassidy for their useful suggestions. And as a truly international project, my gratitude to my researchers and e-mail correspondents: Betty Lawrence in the US, Vikram Naharwar in India and Stephen Peplow in Hong Kong. Producing a book takes time and effort – so my appreciation to all the team at Carlton Books, and my special thanks to photographer, Sue Atkinson and my editor, Richard Emerson for their patience and perfection.

Picture Credits